Praise for Matt Fitzgerald:

"To be a great athlete, you need more than natural ability; you need mental strength to keep going when your body wants to quit. In his new book, writer Matt Fitzgerald dives into the research behind these coping skills and highlights the top athletes who use them. Anyone, whether pro or everyday exercisers, can use these tactics to push further."   —*Men's Journal*

"Fitzgerald has been writing about the psychology of endurance performance for more than a decade now and is really one of the pioneers in terms of trying to take this body of research out of the laboratory and into the field for everyone to try. His latest book examines a series of notable races through the lens of Samuele Marcora's 'psychobiological' theory of endurance. The races make it a fun read, and the psychology is thought-provoking."   —*Runner's World* magazine

"At the highest level of sport, it's often not physiology but psychology that separates the best from the rest. Matt goes well beyond just telling stories of great athletes (though he's really good at doing that, too) and delves deep into cutting-edge brain science to show us all how we can strengthen our own mental muscle."
—Huffington Post, Best Health and Fitness Books in 2015

"This book teaches you how to avoid the many pitfalls of fueling for endurance running and how to use nutrition to improve your performance. I wouldn't marathon without it."
—Jenny Hadfield, author of *Marathoning for Mortals*

"From training day 1 through mile 26.2, Fitzgerald has laid out a nutritional game plan to get you through the wall and to your best marathon yet."   —Desiree Davila, American long-distance runner

"Most nutrition books for athletes are complete garbage. *The New Rules of Marathon and Half-Marathon Nutrition* presents relevant information in a way that is interesting and practical—a fantastic source."

—Brad Hudson, founder and owner of Performance Training Group, coauthor of *Run Faster from the 5K to the Marathon*

"Nutrition is a proven key to success in endurance sports yet the correct approach is often neglected or misunderstood. . . . It is extremely refreshing to see the applications of years of sound sports nutrition spelled out in a precise, comprehensive, and easy-to-read fashion. *The New Rules of Marathon and Half-Marathon Nutrition* is a must-read for beginner and elite-level runners."

—Kimberly Mueller, MS, RD, CSSD, sports dietitian, owner of Fuel Factor Nutrition Coaching, and elite marathoner

"A crucial resource for anyone who wants to run their best marathon. I highly recommend it!"

—Ryan Hall, American record-holder, half marathon and 20K, and Olympian

"Extremely well done. . . . A must for marathoners!"

—*Library Journal*

"You will gain valuable information and insight about how to fuel your body from this book." —*Portland Book Review*

"Written in a friendly and approachable manner and colored with many anecdotal stories from elite running history, this book is an easy and informative read that can help propel your runs to the next level."

—San Francisco/Sacramento Book Review

"I highly recommend reading *Racing Weight* even if you don't need to lose any excess poundage. You'll come away with a better understanding of your physiology and also of food."

—Joe Friel, founder of TrainingBible Coaching and author of *The Triathlete's Training Bible* and *The Cyclist's Training Bible*

"For any triathlete or endurance athlete, or anyone who wonders what it takes to be the best in sport, *Iron War* is an excellent read. . . . Readers will come away with a very strong understanding and appreciation for two of the true legends of our sport . . . as well as a very clear look at the greatest race ever run." —Triathlete.com

"*Iron War* by Matt Fitzgerald recounts the fabled Ironman world championship battle between triathlete legends Dave Scott and Mark Allen. By the end of the story, [triathletes] will feel like [they] personally know the athletes, raced side-by-side with them, and understand the amazing contribution they made to the sport." —Active.com

"The mind is the next frontier for significant performance gains. . . . Mental fitness, says Fitzgerald, means becoming your own sports psychologist and developing coping mechanisms to help you suffer better. Which, while not entirely satisfying, is a good start."

—*Outside Magazine*

"Imagine you could get into the mind of an elite athlete and use their skills to improve your sporting potential. That's the premise of Matt Fitzgerald's *How Bad Do You Want It?*"

—*Triathlon Magazine Canada*

"Fitzgerald is a skilled writer and the drama and excitement of the various races really jump off the pages. If you are feeling a bit unmotivated about running, this would be a *great* book to pick up, as you are likely to be inspired by all of the thrilling stories." —*Run Oregon*

"What better way to reach your goal than with delicious meals designed for weight loss? *Racing Weight Cookbook* delivers 100 recipes targeted for athletes looking to manage their weight."

—*Women's Running* magazine

"If you're looking to get to your peak performance weight or explore the mind–body connection of running, writer Matt Fitzgerald has some advice for you. . . . Fitzgerald, an expert in endurance training and nutrition, explores a wide range of topics and cutting-edge developments from the world of running and endurance sports."

—ESPN.com

"Being a three-time Olympian, I thought I knew all there was to know about diet and training, but Matt blew me away. I can't wait to start implementing all his knowledge into my running."

—Shalane Flanagan, Olympic bronze medalist
and American record-holder

THE ENDURANCE DIET

Also by **Matt Fitzgerald**

How Bad Do You Want It?

Iron War

The New Rules of Marathon and Half-Marathon Nutrition

Racing Weight Cookbook

Racing Weight

Brain Training for Runners

Performance Nutrition for Runners

Diet Cults

80/20 Running

THE ENDURANCE DIET

Discover the **5 CORE HABITS** of the
World's Greatest Athletes to Look,
Feel, and Perform Better

Matt Fitzgerald

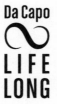

Da Capo

LIFE
LONG

Designed by Amnet Systems
Set in 11.5 point Goudy Std by Perseus Books

Library of Congress Cataloging-in-Publication Data

Names: Fitzgerald, Matt, author.
Title: The endurance diet : discover the 5 core habits of the world's
    greatest athletes to look, feel, and perform better / by Matt Fitzgerald.
Description: First Da Capo Press edition. | Boston, MA : Da Capo Lifelong
    Books, a member of the Perseus Books Group, 2016. | Includes
    bibliographical references and index.
Identifiers: LCCN 2016033907 (print) | LCCN 2016041446 (ebook) | ISBN
    9780738218977 (paperback) | ISBN 9780738218984 (ebook)
Subjects: LCSH: Physical fitness. | Exercise–Physiological aspects. |
    Health. | BISAC: HEALTH & FITNESS / Diets. | HEALTH & FITNESS / Exercise.
Classification: LCC QP301 .F565 2016 (print) | LCC QP301 (ebook) | DDC
    613.7–dc23
LC record available at https://lccn.loc.gov/2016033907

First Da Capo Press edition 2016
ISBN: 978-0-7382-1897-7 (paperback)
ISBN: 978-0-7382-1898-4 (e-book)

Published by Da Capo Press
An imprint of Perseus Books, LLC, a
Subsidiary of Hachette Book Group, Inc.
www.dacapopress.com

Da Capo Press books are available at special discounts for bulk purchases in the U.S. by corporations, institutions, and other organizations. For more information, please contact the Special Markets Department at Perseus Books, 2300 Chestnut Street, Suite 200, Philadelphia, PA, 19103, or call (800) 810-4145, ext. 5000, or e-mail special.markets@perseusbooks.com.

10 9 8 7 6 5 4 3 2 1

CONTENTS

FOREWORD

MOST ATHLETES WOULD AGREE THAT NUTRITION IS IMPORTANT FOR PERFOR-
mance. For endurance athletes, it may be so important that it is the
difference between winning a race and not even making it to the finish
line. When Haile Gebrselassie—who had won pretty much every distance between 1500 and 10,000 meters and set multiple world records
in the process—moved up to the marathon distance, he was facing
Paul Tergat in a show-off at the London marathon. Haile was in top
shape and ready to take on the world . . . who could beat him? It turned
out that poor nutrition beat him. With 12 kilometers to go, he felt his
energy disappearing, his stomach was protesting, and he had to abandon the race. When he figured out his nutrition in the following years,
this did not happen again. Similar mistakes are made by many athletes
with their day-to-day diet.

Although most athletes are aware of the importance of nutrition
and sometimes are even obsessed with their nutrition, very few athletes get it right. In races and training, some athletes overfuel, some
underfuel, some overdrink, some underdrink. A large percentage of
athletes experience gastrointestinal distress, and often these things
are completely preventable. There are multiple reasons why athletes
struggle to get their nutrition right, including (1) not having a plan,
(2) following bad advice, (3) not listening enough to their bodies, (4)
sticking to a plan at all cost, and (5) not being flexible enough with an
existing nutrition plan. People generally think getting nutrition right
is complicated, technical, and difficult to achieve. There is an overload of information and often contradicting advice. Today the general
trend is to remove specific foods from the diet and focus on eating a
smaller number of so-called healthy foods (current popular examples

are the meat-free diet, the low-carb diet, the paleo diet, and many other variations). If foods with little nutritional value are removed and replaced by other more nutritious foods, that may be a good choice. But if the result is that the diet is less diverse, the outcome may not be that positive. Additionally, there are commercial interests, sensationalism, and everyone who writes a blog about nutrition seems to be an expert. It is therefore not surprising that athletes are confused.

As a sports nutrition scientist, I have been at the forefront of research in this field; many of the studies we have done in our labs at the University of Birmingham in the United Kingdom have contributed to the recommendations that we have for athletes to date. My entire career I have tried to translate the sometimes complicated science into practical strategies. Studies are often performed in laboratories so that all variables can be controlled, and this is necessary and it is a good thing. However, laboratories also have a limitation: they are not the same as the training or the races we do. In a lab we can mix a drink using very pure ingredients; in the field we use drinks, products, and foods, and we mix all of them.

The basis of any sensible advice has to be evidence. But this is also exactly the origin of a lot of confusion because people have different views of what evidence is. For some, evidence is a friend who had a good race and says that he took a particular sports drink. For others evidence is a great-looking product they buy at an expo the day before a race. The packaging says "scientifically proven." For me, none of this is evidence. To obtain evidence, a series of rules needs to be followed so that you can establish the actual reason for the good performances.

And that is exactly where Matt Fitzgerald is so brilliant! To distinguish between good and bad science and to separate good and bad communication of science, which is not easy without the specific training and without specific skills, we need people that use their skills to communicate the science and the evidence to the wider audience. Matt is able to read and interpret the science and make it very simple and usable for any athlete. He separates facts from fiction.

In fact, what he communicates may come across as common sense, but that is exactly what is missing sometimes when athletes approach their nutrition.

Matt has researched and explored what elite athletes eat, spending countless hours talking to many of them about their diet. In doing so, he discovered that there are a number of factors that are the same in all the diets of elite endurance athletes all over the world. Many of those athletes had never spoken to a nutritionist, never read about sports nutrition. Yet, their habits have some remarkable similarities.

The Endurance Diet offers the five key nutrition habits Matt has identified, and it turns out that those five common habits are all supported by existing literature and evidence obtained mostly in laboratory studies. And yes, these are elite athletes and they are much faster than the average endurance athlete. But believe it or not, elite athletes are also human. Although there are certainly individual differences, the basic principles of physiology and biochemistry in human bodies are fundamentally the same.

In *The Endurance Diet*, nutrition is brought back to its bare bones. The bells and whistles are removed, the fad diets are broken down, and common sense comes first. I often ask why athletes tend to build their nutrition pyramid starting from the top (often, supplements are the first questions I get from athletes), followed by questions about sports drinks, gels, etc. Far fewer questions are about a balanced healthy diet. This book will help you build the foundation first, well-balanced healthy nutrition, then will help you adapt depending on your activity and your goals.

The beauty is that Matt's endurance diet is not extreme; it is very achievable, it is very sustainable, and it will certainly produce results. Better health as well as better performance. I have found this book to be immensely useful. I hope you will too.

Asker Jeukendrup
Professor of Exercise Metabolism
Loughborough University
Director of mysportscience.com

1 The Diet of the World's Fittest People

WHAT DO PROFESSIONAL RUNNERS IN THE UNITED STATES, NATIONAL-TEAM rowers in Austria, world-class swimmers in Argentina, and champion triathletes in South Africa have in common?

Their diet.

It's true. Elite endurance athletes in every sport and in all parts of the planet eat the same way. Underneath superficial differences in their specific food choices, the world's fittest people share a common set of eating habits that constitute what I call the *Endurance Diet*. Unlike familiar weight-loss and general-health diets, most of which were invented by a single person or group of people, the Endurance Diet evolved over many generations inside the crucible of international competition. Through this process, eating habits that impeded performance were gradually weeded out and only those that best supported it survived.

Yet, although the Endurance Diet is the product of real-world trial and error, not science, the best and latest science demonstrates that its five habits really do maximize the benefits of cardiovascular exercise. A good cardio training program reduces body fat levels, strengthens the heart, improves circulation, increases the body's ability to absorb and adapt to stress, improves metabolic efficiency, sharpens the nervous system, and boosts fatigue resistance in the muscles. These and other physiological adaptations to cardio exercise constitute *endurance fitness*, or the specific type of fitness that elite endurance athletes need to win big races. Studies show that the habits of the Endurance Diet enable athletes to get more endurance fitness out of the same training and also to train more effectively.

Endurance fitness is important not only to elite endurance athletes seeking to win international competitions but also to everyone else who engages in cardio exercise. Endurance fitness is the key to losing weight, improving health, looking better, living longer, functioning and feeling better in everyday life, and achieving any kind of athletic goal, whether it's finishing a half marathon or qualifying for the Ironman World Championship. And the Endurance Diet is the key to maximizing endurance fitness, not just for elite athletes but for everyday athletes and exercisers like us as well.

The only problem is that, although nearly all elite endurance athletes follow the Endurance Diet, very few others do—yet. The purpose of this book is to correct this problem. Whatever form or forms of cardio exercise you may do, and whatever your goal may be, the Endurance Diet will give you better results and a better chance of achieving your goals than any other way of eating. To become as fit as you can be, all you have to do is eat like the world's fittest people. And it's easier than you might think.

Discovering the Endurance Diet

If you're like most endurance athletes and exercisers, you have been exposed to many contradictory claims about what constitutes the optimal diet for endurance fitness. You have probably heard or read that a meat-free diet, a low-carb diet, an ancestral diet, and a host of other diets are best for people seeking endurance fitness. But you probably have *not* heard or read that the diet shared by virtually all of the world's most successful endurance athletes is the way to go. That's because it was only recently discovered that elite endurance athletes all over the world share a common set of eating habits.

The road to this discovery began in 2009, when I was working on a previous diet book for endurance athletes and exercisers. That book included a chapter called "What the Pros Eat," which presented one-day food journals from eighteen of the world's best cross-country skiers, cyclists, mountain bikers, rowers, runners, swimmers, and triathletes.

My reason for incorporating this information was that I believed endurance athletes could not possibly succeed at the highest level unless they ate in a way that supported endurance fitness.

My previous exposure to the diets of elite endurance athletes—going back to 1995, when I wrote an article about the diet of champion triathlete Mike Pigg—had revealed a noteworthy consistency. Almost every world-class performer I'd ever dined with or questioned about his or her eating habits maintained a very balanced and inclusive diet based on natural foods. But the eighteen food journals I collected for my book greatly deepened my appreciation for how similarly top athletes from all over the world nourished themselves. Even some of the same specific menu items—oatmeal, for example—kept popping up.

As I thought about these patterns, I was reminded of the work of Stephen Seiler, an American exercise physiologist who works at the University of Agder in Norway. In the late 1990s, Seiler embarked on a long-term project that entailed rigorously quantifying the training methods of elite endurance athletes in various disciplines. He discovered that world-class athletes in the full suite of endurance sports share a common training approach. Specifically, they spend about 80 percent of their total training time at low intensity and the other 20 percent at moderate to high intensity. Seiler also dug into historical data and learned that elite endurance athletes had not always followed "the 80/20 rule," as he called it. Past generations had experimented with all kinds of methods. But, over the course of many decades, a gradual convergence had occurred.

Seiler has argued persuasively that the reason today's best endurance athletes all train the same way is that the 80/20 approach works better than any alternative. Championship-level competition ruthlessly exposes what works and what doesn't. Athletes who train with superior methods win; athletes who train with inferior methods lose—and then trade their methods for those of the winners. The result is an evolutionary process through which training methods move gradually toward optimal effectiveness.

Having observed that elite endurance athletes from all over the world shared a similar way of eating, I couldn't help but wonder if this pattern did not exist for the same reason elite athletes everywhere had converged on the same training system. It seemed to me more than plausible that the dietary practices that were most broadly shared by elite athletes everywhere were the products of the same type of evolutionary process that had produced their common approach to training, and that these eating habits thus constituted the optimal diet for endurance fitness. I found myself wishing that some ambitious scientist would do the same thing with diet that Seiler had done with training: meticulously examine the eating habits of elite endurance athletes across the globe in order to identify specific practices that are universal within this special group. Then I decided to just go ahead and do it myself.

The research project that I subsequently embarked on took two years to complete. My goal was not to publish the results in a scientific journal for a few dozen PhDs to appreciate but rather to identify a concrete set of best practices for all seekers of endurance fitness to follow. I knew before I even started the project that I would find features common to the diets of most endurance athletes, because I had already seen evidence of their existence. But I hoped to distill the vaguely defined similarities I'd observed previously into a precise, replicable dietary formula, much as Seiler had already done with training.

I spent time eating with and interviewing world-class endurance athletes on five continents. I broke bread with triathletes in Brazil, with cyclists in Spain, with cross-country skiers in Canada, and with Kenyan and Japanese runners. Additionally, I designed a formal diet questionnaire that I sent to world-class athletes in many other countries. A total of thirty-two nations and eleven sport disciplines are represented in the responses I gathered. When my research was complete, I had discovered the Endurance Diet—the optimal diet for endurance fitness.

The Five Key Habits

The Endurance Diet comprises five eating habits that are present in the diets of nearly 100 percent of the athletes I interacted with both directly and indirectly in my research. Expressed in the form of rules, they are as follows:

1. Eat everything
2. Eat quality
3. Eat carb-centered
4. Eat enough
5. Eat individually

These five habits are the final products of a multigenerational process of dietary evolution carried out by elite endurance athletes all over the world, a process in which less effective practices were discarded and more effective practices retained until no further improvement was possible. As such, they represent the necessary and sufficient dietary conditions for attaining the highest possible level of endurance fitness—the rules that today's professional endurance athletes *must* follow in order to win races. Let's take a closer look at what each habit entails and how it benefits the pros who depend on it.

Habit 1: Eat Everything

There are six basic categories of natural whole foods: vegetables (including legumes); fruits; nuts, seeds, and healthy oils; unprocessed meat and seafood; whole grains; and dairy. The overwhelming majority of elite endurance athletes regularly consume all six of these "high-quality" food types. The reason they do so is that a balanced, varied, and inclusive diet is needed to supply the body with everything it needs nutritionally to handle the stress of hard training and to derive the maximum benefit from workouts.

In addition to the six high-quality food types, there are four "low-quality" food types: refined grains, sweets, processed meats, and fried foods. Most elite endurance athletes allow themselves to eat small amounts of each of these food types. Indulging in a treat here and there does them no harm and is even beneficial in the sense that it makes their overall diet more enjoyable and sustainable. (I'll talk in much more detail about food types in Chapters 3 and 4).

Habit 2: Eat Quality

While most elite endurance athletes eat everything, they don't eat equal amounts of everything. Instead they skew their diet heavily toward high-quality foods and eat low-quality foods in moderation. High-quality foods tend to be more nutrient dense (i.e., richer in vitamins, minerals, and antioxidants) and less energy dense (i.e., lower in calories) than low-quality foods. Basing their diet on high-quality foods enables elite endurance athletes to get more overall nutrition from fewer calories, and this in turn allows them to maximize their fitness while maintaining an optimal racing weight.

Habit 3: Eat Carb-Centered

Elite endurance athletes select high-quality carbohydrate-rich foods such as whole grains and fruit as the centerpiece of most meals and snacks. As you probably would expect, there is a great deal of diversity in the specific foods that professional racers from different cultures rely on to meet their carbohydrate needs. Ethiopian runners eat a lot more teff than Chilean mountain bikers, who eat a lot more potatoes than Chinese swimmers, who eat a lot more rice than Danish cross-country skiers. But all of these foods are rich in carbohydrates, and all of these athletes maintain carb-centered diets.

Overall, carbohydrates account for 60 to 80 percent of total calories in the diet of the typical elite endurance athlete. As the primary fuel for intense exercise, carbs enable these athletes to absorb their workouts with less physiological stress and to extract more benefits from their training.

Habit 4: Eat Enough

Elite endurance athletes do not consciously restrict the amount of food they eat by enforcing inflexible calorie counts or portion-size limits or by eating less than is needed to satisfy their hunger, as many recreational athletes and dieters do. Nor do they mindlessly overeat as a majority of people in affluent societies do today. Instead, they pay mindful attention to signals of hunger and satiety and allow these signals to determine when and how much they eat. This is the only reliable way to eat sufficiently but not excessively—that is, enough to meet the energy demands of training but not so much as to gain or hold onto excess body fat.

Habit 5: Eat Individually

Elite athletes are mindful of, and responsive to, not only their appetite but also their dietary needs in general. Each athlete is a unique person in a unique situation. The diet that works best for one athlete is unlikely to work best for another athlete in every detail. For example, while all endurance athletes perform best on a carb-centered diet, some function better when they get most of their carbs from nongrain sources. Elite athletes are good at listening to their bodies, paying attention to how different foods and eating patterns affect them, and modifying their diet according to what they learn. As a result, each professional endurance athlete develops his or her own version of the Endurance Diet.

Among the dozens of elite endurance athletes whose diets I analyzed in my research was Jasmine Alkhaldi, an Olympic swimmer with a Filipino mother and a Saudi father who was competing for the University of Hawaii at the time I interacted with her. Alkhaldi's eating patterns offer a good example of what the Endurance Diet looks like in practice. The table below presents a typical day in her gustatory life.

One-Day Food Journal of Jasmine Alkhaldi, Filipino/Saudi Swimmer
Breakfast: Scrambled eggs with cheese and turkey, old-fashioned oatmeal, banana, coconut water
Snack: Granola bar (whole grains, nuts, seeds), Muscle Milk™ protein shake
Lunch: Grilled fish, quinoa, mixed-greens salad, fruit juice
Dinner: Beef steak, grilled mixed vegetables, fruit juice

All five habits of the Endurance Diet are manifest in this sample day's eating. For starters, it includes each of the six high-quality food types and only one of the four low-quality food types (the Muscle Milk protein shake counts as a sweet). High-carb foods (oatmeal, quinoa, etc.) are the centerpiece of most of her meals and snacks. The frequency and size of her meals are controlled by her appetite, not by calorie counts or plate-cleaning instincts. "I focus on making sure I eat enough because I know I burn all the calories," she explained to me. "I want to make sure that I have something to burn and something that will help my body recover."

Finally, Alkhaldi practices the habit of eating individually by tweaking her diet according to her perception of her body's unique needs. While some elite endurance athletes avoid red meat, for example, Alkhaldi eats it almost daily. "For me personally," she said, "having red meat is a must before any competition because it helps me feel stronger in the water and gain more energy."

The Great Diet Divide

As a certified sports nutritionist, I work one-on-one with nonelite endurance athletes and exercisers who come to me for help with their diet. The most striking thing I've observed in these clients is how few of them eat like the pros before I place them on the Endurance Diet.

The majority of these recreational seekers of endurance fitness instead follow popular diets like the Paleo Diet or else they eat the way the average nonathlete does—which here in the United States, unfortunately, means eating the so-called Standard American Diet (SAD), where 11 percent of total calories come from fast food and 13 percent from added sugars.

Athletes who reach out to me for help are always motivated by a specific problem they're facing, and in almost every case the problem is a direct result of inferior nutrition. The most common problem I see in athletes on the Standard American Diet is difficulty losing weight. But the popular diets, although seemingly healthier, generate negative outcomes, too. After the Paleo Diet became popular, for example, I was contacted by a steady stream of athletes complaining of chronic fatigue and poor performance in workouts.

Why is it that nearly 100 percent of elite endurance athletes like Jasmine Alkhaldi practice all five habits of the Endurance Diet, while most recreational endurance athletes and exercisers do not? The reason has to do with where each group goes for information about how to eat. Elite endurance athletes take their dietary cues from other pros—especially the most successful ones. Nonelite athletes and exercisers, meanwhile, tend to obtain diet information from sources in the mass media and popular culture.

The best athletes do not start off eating differently from the rest of us. In childhood, they (like all of us) eat whatever their parents feed them. Because they are talented, however, they experience great success in their sport even when the food they get at home leaves much to be desired. But when these gifted young athletes finish school and begin to compete against the very best athletes in the world at the professional level, two things happen: (1) they begin to lose races (perhaps for the first time in their life), and (2) they notice that the athletes who are beating them in races eat differently.

The natural response to this situation is also the right one. The defeated younger athletes simply imitate the eating habits of the established winners. Because the overwhelming majority of successful endurance athletes follow the habits of the Endurance Diet, this process invariably consists in the younger athlete adopting any of the five key habits of this diet that he or she is not practicing already. This is how the Endurance Diet perpetuates itself. Having evolved to the point of perfection over the course of many decades, it is now handed down from veteran elite athletes to less experienced ones.

Consider Molly Huddle, one of America's top distance runners. Huddle grew up in Elmira, New York, on what she described to me as "the typical American diet" of cereal for breakfast, sandwiches for lunch, and meat and potatoes for dinner. This diet fueled Huddle to a fourth-place finish at the Foot Locker High School Cross Country Championship and a national high school record for two miles (10:01).

In college, Huddle ate like a typical college athlete. Her dietary mainstays were cold cereal with milk and bagels with peanut butter. Conscious of the need to consume vegetables, she ate salads "occasionally." During her four years at the University of Notre Dame, this diet fueled Huddle to nine All-America selections and a runner-up finish in the 2006 NCAA Championships 5000 meters.

After graduating from college, Huddle moved to Providence, Rhode Island, to train with a group of elite female runners coached by Ray Treacy. Her professional career got off to a shaky start. Huddle struggled initially to keep up with the women she trained with and competed against at the elite level. No longer could she rely on her talent and work ethic alone to dominate her peers. So Huddle decided to change her diet. Wisely, she did not attempt a complete overhaul. She just made a few commonsense adjustments such as eating more salads and less breakfast cereal. In other words, she adopted the Endurance Diet habit of eating quality. The most important change, however, concerned not *what* she ate but *how much*. A naturally light eater, Huddle noticed that the athletes around her ate more, so she began to "eat enough" as well.

"It helped me to see that the women I was training with were eating full, carb-heavy meals and kicking my butt in races," Huddle told me, "so I figured they were doing everything right!"

Her assumption was correct. Running and other endurance sports are so competitive at the elite level today that athletes cannot be successful—no matter how talented and hardworking they are—without doing everything right. They cannot train with inferior methods from yesteryear, use second-rate equipment, or get away with bad dietary habits that affect how their bodies perform in and respond to workouts. Huddle's decision to emulate the eating habits of the best athletes around her just made sense, and it was validated, in the years that followed her dietary adjustments, when she won twenty-three national championship titles and set four American records.

The pattern of Molly Huddle's dietary evolution is extremely common among elite endurance athletes. The only thing that differs from one case to the next is the specific dietary change a given athlete makes at the point of transitioning to the professional level in order to make his or her eating habits conform to the proven best practices of the most successful athletes.

Paweł Ochal is an elite Polish runner with a personal best time of 2:12:20 for the marathon. He comes from a poor family and was raised on an unbalanced diet that contained few fresh fruits and vegetables and no fish whatsoever. After gaining financial support for his running, Ochal greatly increased the variety in his diet. He now eats at least one fruit or vegetable with each meal and snack and spends three months of every year training in Portugal, where he eats fish daily, sometimes twice a day. These improvements have made a marked difference in his body's ability to absorb the training that he must do to be competitive at the pro level and have powered him to successes that include a victory at the Warsaw Marathon.

Stone Tsang, a Chinese adventure racer based in Hong Kong, made an effort to improve the overall quality of his diet as a young professional. He cut down on snack chips and fried food and increased his intake of vegetables, fruit, and nuts. "I've found I feel better and stronger when I eat healthier," he told me.

Dmitry Polyanskiy, a Russian triathlete who finished the 2014 season ranked seventh in the world, grew up on a typical Russian diet.

But when he joined his country's national triathlon team and began to share meals with other elites at training camps, his diet made a significant shift toward carbohydrate-rich foods such as pasta. He discovered that he had a lot more energy for training and racing on a carb-centered eating routine.

Naydene Smith, a South African rower who finished sixth in the 2014 World Rowing Championships Women's Pair, grew up on her mom's home cooking (roasted chicken was a family favorite), but after turning pro she had to modify her diet in a couple of ways to meet her individual needs. She addressed a tendency toward low iron levels with increased red meat consumption and supplementation. Smith also suffers from occasional nondiabetic hyperglycemia, so she is careful to strictly limit her intake of refined sugars.

I could supply many more examples, but these few speak for the rest: Paweł Ochal added balance and variety to his diet (Endurance Diet Habit 1). Stone Tsang elevated the overall quality of his food choices (Endurance Diet Habit 2). Dmitry Polyanskiy increased the amount of carbohydrate in his diet (Endurance Diet Habit 3). Molly Huddle began to make sure that she ate enough (Endurance Diet Habit 4). Naydene Smith adjusted her diet to better meet her individual needs (Endurance Diet Habit 5). These five dietary changes constitute a complete list of the types of dietary changes that elite athletes commonly make in order to excel at the highest level of competition. In each case, the aspiring professional athlete does not abandon the culturally normal diet that he or she grew up on. Instead, a targeted change or set of changes is implemented to make the young athlete's diet more like those of established champions.

Too Much (Mis)Information

Recreational endurance athletes and exercisers like us are in a completely different situation. Unlike the pros, we do not belong to a peer group that clearly has the whole diet thing figured out. For us, discovering the optimal diet for endurance fitness is not a simple matter of copying the eating habits of the Olympians and world champions we train with and compete against. We are left to look for dietary guidance elsewhere. The most popular resources are books, magazines, websites, podcasts, and blogs focused on endurance or general nutrition.

The major drawback of this approach is that the guidance available through such resources is inconsistent. Whereas nearly all elite endurance athletes practice the same five key dietary habits, the authorities offering dietary advice through mass and social media channels have widely varying beliefs about what constitutes the optimal diet for endurance fitness (or weight loss or general health). This lack of consistency leaves many athletes and exercisers confused about what to eat.

A typical case is Kate, a runner in her twenties who works for a nonprofit organization in San Diego. Kate has bounced around from pescatarian to plant-based to other diets and has not been satisfied with any of them. Problems ranging from anemia to severe cravings for "forbidden" foods have caused her to abandon the various eating programs she's tried with initial high hopes. Kate gets much of the information on which she bases her dietary decisions from running websites and publications, but she finds the recommendations they offer to be maddeningly variable.

"I read every running magazine out there," Kate told me. "I've noticed advice given in one issue is completely different than advice in the next issue—and I'm talking about the same publication. How are we supposed to know what is right?"

It's not only twenty-something female runners who are confused about what to eat and whose bewilderment leads them to jump from diet to diet without getting the results they seek. Mike is a fifty-something triathlete who works as a corporate executive in Hoover, Alabama. He has tried high-protein diets, liquid diets, "grazing" diets, and many others. Not an actual client of mine, Mike is still searching. "I have yet to find (or properly execute) a diet where I can successfully manage my weight and feel good in long-distance racing," he told me.

The dietary confusion that endurance seekers feel is exacerbated by the fact that the popular diets they are persuaded to try don't work.

And they don't work to the precise extent that they deviate from the way elite endurance athletes eat.

Most popular diets have rules that contradict one or more of the five habits of the Endurance Diet. Many of them explicitly forbid eating everything. Plant-based diets, which forbid meat, seafood, and dairy, are one example. Popular diets also tend to look past the simple concept of quality in favor of other, more esoteric, ways of distinguishing "good" and "bad" food types, such as glycemic index scores and pH values. A large number of popular diets place strict limits on carbohydrate intake. Others contradict the Endurance Diet habit of eating enough by prescribing calorie counts, portion-size limits, or frequent fasting. And nearly all popular diets at least tacitly discourage individuality, forcing all of their followers to start over with a one-size-fits-all solution instead of allowing them to simply improve their existing (and presumably preferred) eating habits.

Although such rules may sometimes work for people who don't exercise much, they seldom pan out for those who vigorously pursue endurance fitness, regardless of their ultimate goal. I've seen the consequences of each contradiction often enough to have identified consistent patterns.

Dietary Self-Sabotage

Athletes and exercisers who try diets that eliminate entire food groups often come to me with complaints of poor performance in workouts and competitions, compromised recovery, stagnating fitness development, chronic fatigue, injuries, frequent infections, and iron-deficiency anemia. There are also psychological consequences of such restrictions, which include obsessive fear of eating the wrong thing and binge episodes followed by bouts of extreme guilt.

Those who fall for low-carbohydrate diets commonly develop symptoms of overtraining, the worst of which are persistent lethargy, declining performance, hormonal disruptions, and sleep and mood disturbances. Sad to say, the rising popularity of low-carb diets among recreational endurance athletes has been very good for my business as a sports nutritionist.

Athletes and exercisers who approach the task of regulating the amount of food they eat with a negative mind-set, always worrying about gaining weight, usually end up pinballing between overeating and undereating. The latter is just as bad as the former. Consistently falling even slightly short of meeting the athletic body's calorie needs results in poor workout performance, slow recovery between workouts, stagnating fitness, persistent fatigue, mood and sleep disturbances, more frequent illnesses, and elevated risk of injury. There are, of course, many athletes and exercisers who consistently eat too much, but this error is caused not by paying mindful attention to the body's true energy needs, as elite athletes do, but instead by eating low-quality foods that promote overconsumption and by eating "mindlessly" (e.g., cleaning one's plate despite feeling stuffed).

There are also psychological consequences associated with worrying a lot about overeating. Like the mistake of eliminating entire food types from the diet, focusing on not eating too much fosters a fear- and guilt-based relationship with food. I have never met an athlete or exerciser who has an unhealthy relationship with food and yet manages to maintain a consistently healthy diet that produces the desired results.

At the very least, obsessive worry about eating too much causes stress, which sabotages health and fitness as much as healthy food helps it. In the worst cases, this error leads to disordered eating, a problem that is very common at the subelite level of endurance sports and is an outright epidemic among female college runners.

Interestingly, eating disorders are virtually nonexistent among elite endurance athletes. The reason is simple: any elite athlete who develops an eating disorder is not going to stay elite very long! The foundation of endurance fitness is all-around health, and eating enough keeps elite endurance athletes healthy in body and mind.

The most insidious damage that popular diets do to athletes and exercisers results from the discouragement of individuality. A healthy diet is only as effective as it is sustainable. Improved eating habits are more sustainable when they retain some of a person's dietary preferences, but popular diets frequently leave little room for the exercise of such preferences. What's more, one-size-fits-all diets systematically train their followers to ignore their bodies' individual needs, and as a result some of these needs are not met.

For every recreational endurance athlete or exerciser who addresses his or her confusion by cycling through various popular diets, there are several more who react by throwing up their hands and reverting to the Standard American Diet, which has the virtue of being comfortable, at least. One such athlete is Stephanie, a runner and schoolteacher in Linwood, New Jersey, who told me, "I pretty much eat whatever I want, whenever I want, even though I know it's not healthy." Athletes like Stephanie knowingly persist in eating poorly because they are turned off by or burned out on the rigid, perfectionistic popular diets they see as the only alternative to eating "like a normal person," as they often put it.

Features of the SAD have spread well beyond America's borders, so that athletes and exercisers in many parts of the world are now eating too many low-quality foods and not enough high-quality foods. This is one reason why, according to a scientific survey I helped administer in 2008, three out of four recreational endurance athletes report being dissatisfied with their weight at any given time.

Here's Your Opportunity

Chances are you do not currently eat the same way the world's fittest people do. Even if you're not currently following a popular diet or stuck on the Standard American Diet, it is unlikely that you are practicing all five habits of the Endurance Diet like the pros.

This book will give you the opportunity to learn from the world's most successful racers how to eat for maximum endurance fitness. It will give you a virtual seat at the table with top runners, cyclists, and other athletes from a variety of countries so you can see that they do indeed share a common core diet—a diet that works better than any other diet for athletes and exercisers at all levels.

In Chapter 2, I will explain why it makes just as much sense for you to adopt these eating habits as it does for rookie pros like Molly Huddle. Chapters 3 through 7 will supply real-world and scientific proof that these habits are more effective than the alternatives for every endurance fitness seeker, along with specific guidelines on putting them into practice.

The remainder of the book is dedicated to showing you how to make these habits stick and how to fine-tune the Endurance Diet to fit your needs, preferences, and lifestyle. Included in this section is a collection of original recipes for delicious, nourishing, and easy-to-make meals favored by elite endurance athletes all over the world. They were created by Georgie Fear, my longtime collaborator and herself a former triathlete and ultrarunner. The concluding chapter addresses the subject of training, explaining the approach to exercise that best complements the Endurance Diet, the cornerstone of which is Stephen Seiler's 80/20 Rule.

Are you ready for a diet that will cure you once and for all of confusion about how to eat to maximize the results you get from the time and energy you invest in exercise? A diet that will power you beyond all of the nutrition-related obstacles preventing you from achieving your goals? A diet that is as enjoyable and easy to sustain as it is effective because it accommodates individual preferences and needs? Then follow me—or, better yet, follow the athletes who have already gotten where you want to go.

2   Why You Should Eat Like an Elite

AMÄEL MOINARD IS A FRENCH MEMBER OF THE BMC PROFESSIONAL CYCLING team who has completed eleven Grand Tours, including six Tours de France. He is also among the many elite endurance athletes who supplied me with a one-day food journal when I was conducting research on the Endurance Diet.

On the particular day he chose to record his food and beverage intake, Moinard breakfasted on porridge with raisins, banana slices, and soy milk and a cup of tea. He then mounted his bike for a three-hour ride, during which he ate a scone and a cereal bar and drank a bottle of PowerBar Perform and a Coke. Immediately after the ride, Moinard drank a protein shake. His lunch consisted of vegetable-filled strudel with steamed carrots and olive oil and an orange. At midafternoon, he ate an apple and a muffin and drank tea with milk. For dinner, he ate minestrone soup, brown rice, whole wheat bread with butter, and Swiss cheese.

All five habits of the Endurance Diet are manifest in this menu. You will recall from the previous chapter that the first habit is "eating everything," which entails regularly consuming all six of the high-quality food types (vegetables; fruits; nuts, seeds, and healthy oils; unprocessed meat and seafood; whole grains; and dairy) and not forbidding the four low-quality food types (refined grains, sweets, processed meats, and fried foods). Moinard's food journal includes every food type except fried foods and unprocessed/processed meat and seafood. Moinard explained to me that he consumes meat or fish every other day. If he had recorded his food journal one day earlier or one day later than he actually did, we would have seen meat or fish on his dinner plate.

Habit 2 is "eating quality." This means basing your diet on the high-quality food types and eating only small amounts of the low-quality food types. Most of the low-quality foods and drinks recorded in Moinard's food journal were taken in during exercise, when the normal rules of healthy eating are suspended, for the simple reason that the purpose of consuming nutrition during exercise is to enhance performance, not health, and the most performance-enhancing forms of nutrition you can consume during exercise are sports drinks and other high-sugar products that are not healthy to consume outside of exercise. The only low-quality foods Moinard ate in the context of regular meals and snacks were strudel and a muffin (both made with refined grains) and milk chocolate (a sweet).

The third habit of the Endurance Diet is "eating carb-centered." Practicing this habit is a matter of putting carbohydrate-rich foods at the center of most meals and snacks. Moinard certainly did so on this day, eating porridge and a banana at breakfast, taking in lots of carbs on the bike, eating strudel at lunch and brown rice and bread at dinner, and snacking on fruit. Over the course of the full day, Moinard got more than 70 percent of his total calories from carbs (including nutrition taken in on the bike).

Habit 4, "eating enough," consists of regulating the amount of food that you eat by paying mindful attention to, and heeding, internal signals of hunger and satiety. Athletes who do so eat enough to maximize the benefits of their training without overeating. The alternatives to mindful eating are restricted eating (e.g., counting calories), which tends to result in yo-yoing between undereating and compensatory overeating, and mindless eating (e.g., plate cleaning), which tends to result in consistent overeating.

It is not possible to discern from a food journal whether an athlete eats mindfully, but it is possible to quantify how much he eats, and it's clear from Amäel Moinard's food journal that he eats a lot. There are six separate eating occasions recorded in his journal, and even the snacks are substantial. Nothing less would have sufficed to meet his energy needs. Moinard burned more than 5,000 calories on the day in question. But he did not meet his energy needs by consciously limiting himself to 5,000 calories. Instead he ate by feel, taking in just enough food to satisfy his appetite and stave off the return of hunger until it was time to eat again.

The fifth habit is "eating individually." This entails applying the other four habits in a way that accommodates an athlete's individual needs and preferences. Like Habit 4, this one is all about paying attention to yourself. But whereas eating enough results from eating mindfully, eating individually results from the somewhat broader practice of eating consciously, or paying attention to how your body responds to various eating patterns and adjusting them to enhance positive outcomes and eliminate negative outcomes.

Moinard's practice of alternate-day vegetarianism is a great example of eating individually. It's not something that many elite endurance athletes do, but Moinard has found that when he eats meat and fish more often, he gains weight, whereas if he eats them less often, he loses power on the bike.

Another elite endurance athlete who supplied me with a one-day food journal is Gwen Jorgensen, an American triathlete who won the ITU Triathlon Series World Championship in 2014 and 2015 and the 2016 Olympic Women's Triathlon. Despite living in a different country and competing in a different sport than Amäel Moinard, she maintains a diet that is very similar to his.

The breakfast Jorgensen recorded in her food journal consisted of a bowl of oatmeal with banana slices, raisins, goji berries, strawberries, nuts, coconut oil, yogurt, peanut butter, and two poached eggs; coffee; and a piece of dark chocolate. After her first workout, she ate a snack of rice cakes with peanut butter and Greek yogurt. Lunch consisted of steamed rice with lamb and vegetables and a second piece of dark chocolate. Following her afternoon workout, Jorgensen ate dried apples, hummus, and raisins. Dinner was a one-pot dish with sweet potato, veggies, chicken, feta cheese, and avocado. Dessert was another piece of dark chocolate. Before going to bed, Jorgensen snacked on muesli with yogurt and fruit.

Perhaps the most striking feature of this menu is the sheer volume of food Jorgensen ate. If she's not practicing the habit of eating enough, I'm Santa Claus! Almost as striking are the variety and balance of Jorgensen's diet. Her food journal includes three servings of vegetables, four servings of fruit, four servings of nuts, seeds, and healthy oils, two servings of whole grains, three-and-a-half servings of dairy, and four servings of unprocessed meat and seafood (including the poached eggs). Clearly, she is fully on board with the habit of eating everything.

Almost all of the variety in Jorgensen's food selections comes from the six high-quality food categories. The only exceptions are the two servings of white rice she ate (one in the form of rice cakes) and her second and third squares of dark chocolate (the first one deserves a pass, as research indicates that dark chocolate is healthy in small amounts).

Like Moinard, Jorgensen puts high-carb foods at the center of each meal and snack, from the oatmeal she consumes almost every day at breakfast to the muesli she ate before bedtime on this particular day. And like Moinard again, Jorgensen permits herself a few dietary eccentricities that demonstrate a habit of eating individually. For example, lots of people add fruit and nuts to their oatmeal, as Jorgensen does. But not many also add coconut oil, yogurt, peanut butter, and poached eggs! Jorgensen created this unusual breakfast dish as a way to get the dietary variety and balance she feels her body needs.

No Coincidence

The fact that Amäel Moinard and Gwen Jorgensen's diets are so similar would hold no real significance if other elite endurance athletes did not eat similarly. But in fact nearly all of the professional racers whose diets I have analyzed practice all five habits of the Endurance Diet.

Even this broader pattern would mean little, however, if most recreational endurance athletes and exercisers and even nonathletes throughout the world practiced the same habits. If this were the case, then the Endurance Diet would be nothing more than the way everyone eats. But data from large-scale scientific surveys and from epidemiological research clearly shows that few people other than professional endurance racers practice all five habits of the Endurance Diet.

What's more, even elite endurance athletes themselves did not follow the Endurance Diet. Looking at what earlier generations of elite endurance athletes put into their mouths, we find that they deviated from one or more of the five habits far more often than today's athletes do. Here are some notable examples:

- The first great runner of the twentieth century, Hannes Kolehmainen, who lived from 1889 to 1966, did not practice the habit of eating everything. He was, in fact, a vegetarian.

- Johnny Weissmuller, the greatest swimmer of the 1920s, did not eat quality. He survived mainly on hot dogs and ice cream and consumed few vegetables except when his coach was looking over his shoulder.

- Jacques Anquetil, who won the Tour de France five times between 1957 and 1964, did not eat a lot of carbohydrates. He was raised on the high-fat, dairy-rich diet of working-class Normandy, which he supplemented as an adult professional cyclist with copious amounts of protein-packed steak and lobster as well as vast quantities of champagne (alcohol is not a carb!).

- Peter Reid, a Canadian triathlete who won the Ironman World Championship three times between 1998 and 2003, did not eat enough. A big man by the standards of world-class triathletes, Reid sometimes went to bed at night so hungry that he had a headache, all for the sake of getting down to what he considered to be his ideal racing weight of 164 pounds.

- Wang Junxia, a Chinese runner who set a women's 10,000-meter world record in 1993, did not eat individually, adjusting her diet to meet her personal needs and preferences. Junxia was trained by an infamously despotic coach named Ma Junren, who ruled his all-female roster of athletes with an iron fist, micromanaging every aspect of their lives, diet included. Although he allowed them to eat some normal foods, like rice, he also forced them to consume turtle's blood, caterpillar fungus, and other supplements with supposed endurance-boosting powers.

Taken together, these three facts—(1) that nearly all elite endurance athletes today share the same five key eating habits, (2) that most recreational endurance athletes and exercisers and most sedentary people do not practice all of these same habits, and (3) that elite endurance athletes of past generations were far more likely than today's top racers to disobey one or more of the "rules" of the Endurance Diet—demand an explanation. Why did this way of eating evolve to become almost universal at the top level of every major endurance sport while remaining uncommon elsewhere?

Survival of the Fittest

The short answer is *competition*. Endurance races like the Boston Marathon and the Ironman World Championship determine winners and losers with brutal clarity. The rewards for winning these competitions—money, fame, glory, and the thrill of victory itself—are significant and function as strong incentives for athletes to do everything in their power to cross the finish line first.

Most races are won by the fittest participant. Technique and tactics matter less in endurance competition than they do in games like tennis and soccer, while fitness matters more. The fittest athlete on the start line of a race is very likely to be the first one to cross the finish line, even if he or she is not the best tactician and does not have the most refined technique. In a sense, then, most races are decided before they even start. The true challenge for elite endurance athletes, therefore, is to arrive at the start line with the highest level of fitness.

The three main contributors to fitness are talent, training, and diet. Talent, of course, is fixed at birth, whereas training and diet are controllable and are thus the focus of each athlete's efforts to prepare for competition. In a race contested by athletes of equal talent, the fittest participant and the probable winner will be the one who is best prepared, and the one who is best prepared will be the one who trained and ate in the most effective ways before the race.

If there were only one way to train or eat, then almost every race would be won by the most talented athlete. But in fact there is an almost infinite variety of ways to train and eat in preparation for endurance competition. Knowing this, and knowing the importance of training and diet to fitness, elite athletes who fall short of victory in major races often try to find out how the winners train and eat and then imitate those practices.

The history of endurance sports is filled with examples of such copy-catting. Consider the case of Finnish runners Hannes Kolehmainen (mentioned above) and Paavo Nurmi. In 1912, Kolehmainen won Olympic gold medals in three running events and became a national hero. In the wake of these triumphs, thousands of Finnish boys took up running in the hope of becoming their country's next athletic icon. Many of these young runners also emulated the specific methods that were perceived as the secrets to Kolehmainen's success.

There were two salient ways in which Kolehmainen's methods of preparing for competition differed from the methods used by most of his contemporaries. On the training side, Kolehmainen was innovative in his use of high-intensity intervals. On the diet side, he stood out as a vegetarian. Paavo Nurmi was fifteen years old when the Summer Games of 1912 were staged in Stockholm. He took up running and became a vegetarian the very same year. For whatever reason, though, he did not immediately incorporate high-intensity intervals into his training routine. After showing initial promise, Nurmi struggled to improve. Then, at age twenty-one, he gave up vegetarianism and started doing high-intensity intervals. Soon thereafter, Nurmi experienced a breakthrough, lowering his 5000-meter time by 32 seconds and qualifying for the 1920 Olympics in Antwerp, where he won the 10,000 meters and the individual cross country event and led Finland to the team cross country title.

This example perfectly illustrates how the evolution of training methods and dietary practices has occurred at the elite level in endurance sports. Most of the major endurance sports can trace their origins to the late nineteenth century. (The first European Rowing

Championship was held in 1893, for example, and the first Olympic Marathon in 1896.) Among the first few generations of modern endurance athletes, training methods and dietary practices were extremely diverse and constantly changing. But as up-and-coming athletes like Paavo Nurmi emulated champions like Hannes Kolehmainen, an evolutionary process began to unfold.

Not everything that the champions did differently was necessarily better. In those early days, exceptionally talented athletes were able to win despite making mistakes. But things sorted themselves out over time, as up-and-comers with varying degrees of talent tested out training methods and dietary practices borrowed from the champions. Some methods and practices, such as high-intensity intervals, proved to be effective for everyone, whereas others, such as vegetarianism, proved to be less effective than a specific alternative (in this case eating everything).

As the decades passed, two things happened. First, there was a gradual convergence of the training methods and dietary practices used by elite endurance athletes all across the world. At the same time, the top racers got fitter and faster—proof that this evolutionary process was moving elite athletes inexorably toward optimal, unimprovable ways of preparing. Kolehmainen's best time for 5000 meters was 14:36.6. The *women's* world record at that distance now stands at 14:11.5.

Each of the five habits of the Endurance Diet traveled its own path toward universality within the elite athlete population. Prioritizing carbohydrates in the diet, for example, has been the norm since the 1960s. Eating quality, on the other hand, did not become universal until more recently. The most dominant marathoner of the late 1970s, Bill Rodgers, for example, had a notoriously junk-filled diet.

There is compelling evidence that it is no longer possible for even the most extraordinarily talented athlete to win major international competitions despite defying one or more habits of the Endurance Diet. Consider the case of Peter Reid, the three-time Ironman champion who defied the Endurance Diet habit of eating enough. Only once since Reid won his last Ironman title in 2003 has the winning time of that event been slower than Reid's best winning time. Two of those faster victories were achieved by Chris McCormack, who weighed 177 pounds, or 13 pounds more than the weight that Reid starved himself down to for race day. Notably, McCormack's first Ironman win came in the Australian's sixth attempt, and he'd been as light as 171 pounds in some of his previous attempts. Only when he stopped worrying about being as light as possible and started to eat enough did McCormack break through to victory.

What's true of the habit of eating enough as it relates to the Ironman World Championship is also true of the other four Endurance Diet habits and for every other major international endurance sports race. Over the past 120 years, the crucible of championship-level competition, by rewarding superior fitness and mercilessly punishing its lack, has led elite endurance athletes to discover the very best way to eat for endurance fitness. Athletes who do not eat this way simply cannot win at the highest level.

The Science of Trial and Error

We have just seen convincing historical evidence that the Endurance Diet is in fact the optimal diet for endurance fitness. But historical evidence is not scientific proof. Nowadays, people expect diets to have a scientific basis. Can we really trust that a real-world process of blind trial and error enabled elite endurance athletes to discover the diet that supports endurance fitness better than any other way of eating?

Why not? Trial and error solves all kinds of real-world problems. Most notably, natural selection, which influences how living species survive in challenging and changing environments, is a form of trial and error. Natural selection parallels the process by which the Endurance Diet evolved in the environment of elite endurance competition. Like endurance athletes, animals, plants, and other living species seek *fitness*—not endurance fitness, in their case, but the fitness of being well adapted to their environment. The individual members of a living species have different physical traits that confer varying degrees of fitness in relation to their environment. Each trait represents a distinct potential solution to the problem of the species' survival. These traits are the functional equivalent of the various training methods and dietary practices that athletes use to pursue endurance fitness.

Whereas endurance athletes compete for race victories, organisms compete to procreate. Individual organisms whose traits render them better adapted to their environment are more likely to live long enough to produce offspring. Consequently, favorable traits tend to spread throughout a species over succeeding generations, whereas unfavorable traits tend to get weeded out.

The trial-and-error approach to problem solving—whether the problem is the survival of a species in a changing environment or discovering the optimal diet for endurance fitness—is essentially a form of random guessing. The downside of random guessing is that it's inefficient. Consider how long it would take you to guess a randomly chosen number between one and one million (unless you got incredibly lucky). The upside of trial and error is that, given enough time, it's guaranteed to succeed. As biophysicist John Mayfield wrote in his book, *The Engine of Complexity*, "Random guessing will eventually answer any question." If you're given a million chances to guess a randomly chosen number between one and one million, you can't possibly fail.

There are far more than one million combinations of dietary patterns that could conceivably combine to define the optimal diet for endurance fitness. The human body produces an estimated 2,709 enzymes that facilitate approximately 896 chemical reactions. In athletes, all of these enzymes and reactions serve as direct or indirect links between diet and fitness. Each specific change in diet—for example, altering the ratio of cooked foods to raw foods that are consumed—has the potential to influence this complex biochemistry in ways that may in turn affect endurance fitness. A very large number of "random guesses" are therefore needed to answer the question of how to eat for maximum endurance fitness.

Not an infinite number, however. The past 120-plus years have given elite endurance athletes around the world enough opportunity to test just about every possible solution to the problem of how to eat for maximum endurance fitness. The fact that, after fourteen or so generations, elite athletes across all disciplines and on every continent have settled on a common solution assures us there is little left to try.

Does this mean that science has no role to play in identifying the optimal diet for endurance fitness? Not at all. Sports nutritionists and exercise physiologists contribute to the process by testing the relative effectiveness of different dietary practices in a more formal and focused way than real-world racing does. Research of this kind has consistently demonstrated that Endurance Diet habits yield better results than the alternatives, and that the various popular diets often followed by recreational endurance athletes fail to live up to their promises.

A good example is the Zone Diet. The creator of the Zone Diet, Barry Sears, was working as a biochemist when he came across a scientific paper that caught his interest. In it, Sanford Byers and Meyer Friedman of Mount Zion Medical School in San Francisco reported that they had reversed symptoms of atherosclerosis in rabbits by injecting them with phospholipids, a type of fat used mainly in cell membranes.

Several years later, Sears learned of new research on a class of molecules called eicosanoids, which are synthesized from phospholipids and participate in many biological functions, including inflammation. This new research convinced Sears that eicosanoids were much more important than he had previously known. Many years later he wrote, "These hormones . . . are among the most powerful and important substances in the body. They act as 'master switches' that control virtually all human body functions. . . . Eicosanoids are so crucial to our health and well-being that I came to think of them as the 'molecular glue' that holds the human body together."

Having come to this conclusion, Sears set out to discover a way to balance eicosanoids for maximum health. This mission led eventually to his development of the Zone Diet. The original version of the diet offered a very simple prescription: get 40 percent of your daily calories from carbohydrates and 30 percent each from fat and protein. A later iteration of the program introduced an element of essential fatty acid supplementation. Sears brought the Zone Diet to the masses with his first book, *Enter the Zone*, which was published in 1995 and became an international bestseller. The Zone Diet gained popularity with recreational endurance athletes after Sears licensed the 40-30-30 concept to a sports supplement company that incorporated the formula into a line of energy bars and marketed them aggressively to athletes.

Although the Zone Diet was not created for endurance athletes, Barry Sears was able to create a *post factum* argument to support the idea that it was optimal for endurance fitness nevertheless. Specifically, he argued that his diet increased the body's production of particular eicosanoids involved in muscle growth and repair, blood flow and muscle oxygenation, and inflammation. If eicosanoids truly were as all-important as Sears contended, this argument probably would have stood up to formal testing. But in a 2002 study, researchers at England's Kingston University found that switching over to the Zone Diet *reduced* running performance by almost 10 percent in a group of moderately fit young men.

One of the reasons the Zone Diet became so popular among recreational endurance athletes was that it *seemed* so scientific. But there's a difference between seeming scientific and being scientific. A biochemical explanation for why a certain diet *ought* to maximize endurance fitness should not be mistaken for proof that it does. And if that biochemical explanation is based on just one or two small pieces of the huge and complex puzzle of human metabolism—such as eicosanoids, which do not, in fact, "act as 'master switches' that control virtually all human body functions" and are not, in fact, "the 'molecular glue' that holds the human body together"—then it really isn't much better than a random guess. A stronger hypothesis would have to consider the complete metabolic puzzle—all of the human body's estimated 2,709 enzymes and 896 chemical reactions—and that is simply impossible. It's better just to skip the hypothesizing and revert to trial and error, a process that, thankfully, has already been fully played out in the real world.

Other popular diets that are followed by endurance athletes have similar flaws. Proponents of plant-based diets, high-fat diets, and other regimens offer very scientific-seeming biochemical explanations for why they *ought* to maximize endurance fitness. But like Barry Sears's case for the Zone Diet, these explanations are nothing more than highly reductionistic stories of "biological plausibility"—wild guesses dressed up in the language of biochemistry—so it shouldn't be surprising at all that, when actually put to the test, these guesses turn out to be wrong.

But although human metabolism is just too complex to allow scientists to deduce the optimal diet for endurance fitness through biochemistry, science can, in addition to testing the effectiveness of different dietary practices in a more formal and focused way than races do, shed light on why the most effective practices work and why the least effective ones don't. For example, recent research indicates that the problem with the Zone Diet is that it's too high in protein. (To meet the 30 percent protein requirement of the Zone Diet, the average American would have to almost double his or her protein intake, and the average American's diet is already high in protein by global standards.) A 2013 study by Japanese scientists found that eating a lot of protein inhibits the development of endurance fitness by reducing the number of mitochondria—the little "factories" inside muscle cells where aerobic metabolism occurs—that the body creates in response to training. This is not to say that 30 percent protein is "bad"—in fact, as I will discuss in Chapter 9, it's actually good for short-term weight loss—it's just not good for building endurance fitness.

In the coming chapters I will share much more scientific proof that the Endurance Diet habits are essential to maximizing endurance fitness, as well as research showing how these habits work. But the most persuasive argument in favor of these habits is the real-world evidence we've already seen: winners use them.

We're All Human

In 2015, I gave a presentation titled "Why You Should Eat Like an Elite" (sound familiar?) at a summit for running coaches. Halfway through my talk, an audience member raised a hand and said, "I don't get it. Elite athletes are completely different from the people I coach. How can the diet of an Olympic champion possibly apply to someone who runs a 25-minute 5K?"

It was a fair question, and perhaps one that has crossed your mind as well. If so, I'm glad, because it means I've probably succeeded in convincing you that the Endurance Diet is at the very least the optimal diet for *elite* endurance athletes. But does it really work for everyone?

Here's what I told that skeptical coach: Elite endurance athletes aren't as different from the rest of us as you might think. DNA analyses have demonstrated that a mere handful of genes, such as certain variants of the FIF5B gene, distinguish Olympic champions from the average Joe and Jane. Most of these genes relate to body size, natural speed, and aerobic capacity. They have nothing to do with how food is digested and metabolized.

Nor, for that matter, do these genes have anything to do with how the body responds to training. Scientists have determined that the genes that confer the ability to gain aerobic fitness in response to training (or "trainability") are quite widespread in the human population. In one study, exercise physiologists created a system for scoring trainability based on how many of the relevant genes a person had. Although there was a significant degree of interindividual variation, a greater number of subjects (52) had the highest possible score than the lowest (36).

Recreational endurance athletes and exercisers typically do not train nearly as much as the pros do, and it is widely assumed that most of them couldn't match elite training volumes even if they wanted to. But genetic findings like those I just described indicate that a majority of nonelite endurance athletes actually could get much fitter if they emulated the high-volume training of the pros.

Running is a bit of an exception. Most recreational runners could not handle 120 miles of running per week. But this limitation is mainly related to body size, not trainability. Recreational runners tend to be much larger than the pros (the current world record holder in the men's marathon is five-foot-seven and weighs 121 pounds), and therefore their bodies absorb much more impact force with each mile, causing greater wear and tear.

Another popular assumption is that recreational athletes can and should "make up for" training less than the elites by doing more of their training at high intensity. This assumption is also false. Studies have shown that recreational athletes who exercise less than 45 minutes a day, on average, get the best results when they spend 80 percent of that time at low intensity and 20 percent at moderate to high intensity, just like the elites.

The science is clear: elite and recreational endurance athletes are similar enough physiologically that the training methods that work best for the pros are also most effective for the rest of us.

And diet? Some proponents of popular diets for endurance athletes have proposed that recreational athletes and exercisers, because they do not train as much as the elites, cannot "get away with" eating as the elites do. These Endurance Diet skeptics see habits such as eating everything, eating carb-centered, and eating enough as forms of dietary laxness that require several hours of daily training to neutralize. But elite athletes don't practice these habits because they *can*—they practice them because they *must*.

If the goal of elite athletes were merely to look good naked, many of them could eat fast food three times a day and still maintain their washboard stomachs by virtue of burning thousands of calories a day through exercise. But elite athletes are trying to achieve something far more difficult than looking good naked—they are trying to win major international competitions. To achieve this goal, they need to be significantly leaner and fitter than they would have to be merely to *look* lean and fit. Therefore, they cannot afford to have any true laxness in their diet.

A 2009 study involving elite runners drives this point home. Twenty-one top-level Ethiopian milers—ten women and eleven men—were statistically lined up in the order of their best race times. All of these athletes were very fast, but some were marginally faster than others. In a second part of the experiment, the same runners were statistically lined up in the order of their body fat percentage. All of them were very lean, but some were just slightly leaner than others. As it turned out, the two lineups—the speed-based arrangement and the fat-based arrangement—were almost identical. The fastest runner among the twenty-one was also the leanest, the second fastest was the second leanest, and so forth.

These findings make it clear that elite endurance athletes do not have any margin to "get away with" sloppy eating habits. Whatever may appear like sloppiness to some—such as eating lots of carbs—is actually necessary to attain the razor-thin advantages that separate winners from losers at the elite level.

It is interesting to see what happens when an elite athlete whose diet really is substandard—meaning it does not fully conform to the five habits of the Endurance Diet—brings it up to standard at midcareer. One such case involves the American triathlete Hunter Kemper. Through the first several years of his professional career, Kemper was a somewhat careless eater with a weakness for Krispy Kreme donuts. Despite this weakness, Kemper performed very well, winning three national championship titles between 1998 and 2004 and finishing as high as eighth in the world championships—and he certainly *looked* lean and fit. But he wanted more.

After a disappointing ninth-place finish at the 2004 Olympics in Athens, Kemper decided to make some changes. He consulted with a sports nutritionist and subsequently improved his diet quality by eating more vegetables and unprocessed meats and fewer donuts and other sweets. He lost a couple pounds of hidden body fat and finished the 2005 season as the ITU World Cup champion and the number-one ranked triathlete in the world.

Recreational endurance athletes with far less talent and significantly milder training schedules than Hunter Kemper achieve similar results when they make similar changes. Take Cassandra, a formerly overweight fifty-something triathlete and network specialist from Spokane, Washington. Cassandra used my Diet Quality Score tool (which I'll describe in Chapter 4) to improve her diet and subsequently lost 110 pounds without making any other changes to her eating or exercise habits. "It was pretty easy to drop the weight without 'dieting' or adversely affecting my triathlon training," she told me via Facebook.

As you see, the eating habits that work best for athletes at one end of the talent and training spectrum really do work just as well for athletes and exercisers at the opposite end. It's a simple fact: if you want to become as healthy and fit as you can be given the amount of time you're able to invest in your training, you need to eat like an elite.

3   Habit 1: Eat Everything

IN THE WINTER OF 2015 I TRAVELED FROM MY HOME IN CALIFORNIA'S CEN-
tral Valley to the Spanish resort village of Mojácar Playa to spend a
few days with the LottoNL-Jumbo professional bike racing team. I met
the cyclists at the Hotel Marina Playa, a four-star accommodation situated fifty meters from a private beach on the Mediterranean Sea and
equipped with four pools, indoor and outdoor bars, a golf course, a
full-service spa, and racquet courts. The mostly Dutch athletes were
not there to enjoy such amusements, however. They had come for
a ten-day training camp, and their attitude was all business, for the
stakes were high.

Earning a position on a World Tour cycling team like LottoNL-Jumbo
is about as difficult as making the roster of a Major League Baseball
team. Holding on to such a position isn't any easier. Most of the
twenty-five members of the LottoNL-Jumbo team are on one- or two-
year contracts. Each rider must consistently perform well in races to get
his contract renewed. And a rider must first prove himself in training
before he is even given the opportunity to represent the team in the
bigger races. (Only nine men are selected for the Tour de France, for
example.) The proving process begins with the team's annual late January training camp on Spain's southeastern coast.

The team's managers are under no less pressure than its athletes.
Only eighteen teams are selected annually by the Union Cycliste Inter-
nationale (the international governing body of the sport of cycling) to
participate in the World Tour, which comprises the twenty-eight pre-
mier international cycling events. A team that makes the cut one year
will be left out the next if its riders fail to perform.

In short, everything depends on results, and results, in turn, depend on doing everything right, beginning with training and diet. A substantial portion of Lotto's resources, therefore, are devoted to regulating the riders' eating. In Mojácar Playa, support staff outnumbered athletes eighteen to sixteen (the other nine riders were racing in Australia), and a third of those staff members served in nutrition-related capacities. Nutritionist Marcel Hesseling planned all of the riders' meals. Team chef Jesper Boom prepared the meals with the help of his assistant, Marije Hengeveld. Frank van Eerd was responsible for the baking. Van Eerd owns and operates a specialty bakery in Holland but is contracted to supply the team's bread products. ("We Dutch take our bread *very* seriously," he told me.) Also in Spain were Gerard Rietjens, an exercise physiologist who plans and executes much of the testing that leads to adjustments in the team's fueling practices, and Louis Delahaije, who bears the title of "high-performance manager" and does wide-ranging research in pursuit of better ways to nourish the riders.

The Hotel Marina Playa has a large buffet of decent quality. The cost of eating three meals a day there is included in the price of a room at the resort. It would have been convenient and cost effective for the LottoNL-Jumbo riders to have relied on the buffet to fill their bellies throughout the training camp. But they did not. Instead, the team shipped two pallets of their own food from Holland.

One of LottoNL-Jumbo's sponsors is a Dutch food service called Daily Fresh, which prepares high-quality fresh meals in small portions and then vacuum seals them at their facility for quick and easy reheating wherever the team happens to be. The riders get all of their hot meals in Daily Fresh form during races. One of the benefits of this system is that it virtually eliminates the risks of food poisoning and of consuming foods tainted with substances (such as certain steroids used on livestock) that might trigger a positive result in a doping test. Another benefit is that it gives the team management an extremely high degree of control over what goes into the riders' bodies. In Spain, the team did not rely on this system quite as heavily as it does at races.

Hot entrees from Daily Fresh were supplemented with fresh produce and breakfast foods brought from Holland and with select items from the buffet.

The team took their meals in a medium-size room called the "Sala Oriente" that was situated just off the main dining area. My first meal with the athletes was a Saturday breakfast, served at eight o'clock. This was the one meal of the day for which Chef Boom did not prepare a special menu, instead supplying the riders with a selection of staple items available at every breakfast. These included cereals, breads, and crepes made by Frank van Eerd, a variety of spreads, and fresh fruit. Athletes who wanted hot items other than the crepes could get them from the buffet.

Steven Kruijswijk, a twenty-seven-year-old racer whose palmarès included an eighth-place finish at the 2011 Giro d'Italia, mixed plain yogurt, whole-grain granola with raisins and currants, whey protein powder, and banana slices in a big bowl and gobbled it up. He rounded out the meal with several orange wheels and a generous blob of cottage cheese, washing it all down with a cup of unsweetened tea. Maarten Wynants, a thirty-two-year-old cyclist who took tenth place at Paris-Roubaix in 2012, ate a whole-grain spelt crepe with apple butter, a plain one-egg omelet, and a few pieces of whole-grain bread, one covered with peanut butter, another with Nutella, and one or two more with marmalade honey. He drank coffee.

It was an important meal for all of the athletes. Later that morning they would complete their first major fitness test of the 2015 season. Their performance in this workout would provide the coaches with crucial data that would influence their decisions concerning early season racing opportunities. Many of the athletes were as nervous as they would have been before an actual race.

I got into a team car with Louis Delahaije and Gerard Rietjens and was driven to the top of the mountain where the testing was to take place. The cyclists took the scenic route to the base of the mountain, arriving there after two full hours in the saddle. At that point the riders were sent off individually at one-minute intervals. They were instructed to climb steadily for six minutes, stopping when they reached the spot where the team car was parked. Delahaije and Rietjens would then take a tiny blood sample from a fingertip and measure its concentration of lactate, a metabolic marker of exercise intensity. The coaches would also collect heart rate and power output data from the rider before freeing him to pedal back down the mountain, turn around, and climb again. The athletes would complete a total of six climbs, pushing a little harder each time and going all-out in the final ascent.

Throughout the ride, the cyclists fueled themselves with energy gels and sports drinks; if the workout had been longer and less intense, they would have gotten less of their energy from such products and more from real foods, including homemade energy bars made with fruit and whole grains by Frank van Eerd.

From our vantage, we could see the riders negotiating the switchbacks most of the way up. At the starting point they appeared as tiny splotches of yellow. It seemed incredible to me that in just six minutes they were able to climb all the way to where we waited. Several of the riders sustained outputs exceeding 500 watts on the last climb, enough power to have propelled them at nearly 35 mph for more than three miles on a flat road.

When the test was complete, the riders returned to the hotel, taking the short way this time. The total duration of the ride was a little under four hours. As soon as the cyclists dismounted, they were handed bottles containing a whey protein drink. They then showered and went straight to the Sala Oriente for a late (3:00 p.m.) lunch. Chef Boom had prepared a diverse banquet centered on a pair of hot entrees: a lasagna and whole-grain focaccia topped with cheese, olives, and other goodies.

LottoNL-Jumbo team leader Laurens ten Dam, a climbing specialist who finished ninth in the 2014 Tour de France, ate both entrees and a large garden salad with tomatoes, celery, and peppers plus a few slices of cold roast beef. For dessert he chose melon slices and pineapple chunks. He drank water and coffee, and, just before leaving the Sala, he made a small turkey sandwich to eat later. Sep Vanmarcke, a rising star who took second at Paris-Roubaix in 2013, skipped the lasagna, added pine nuts to his salad, chose turkey slices instead of roast beef, and finished the meal with yogurt. On the way out he grabbed one of van Eerd's homemade energy bars.

After lunch, the athletes took turns visiting the rooms of the team soigneurs for massages. These rooms were well stocked with snacks: bananas, golden raisins, grapes, gummies, muesli, oranges, pretzel sticks, protein shakes, snack bars, soy milk, trail mix, and yogurt. Whether or not the riders availed themselves of any of these items, at 5:30 in the afternoon all of them were given a smoothie made with avocado, banana, honey, and yogurt to drink.

The Spanish eat dinner late, a custom that suited team Lot-toNL-Jumbo just fine on this day. At 8:00 the riders were again seated in the Sala Oriente. On Chef Boom's menu was a salad of mixed greens with broccoli florets, beets, goat cheese, and pine nuts; ratatouille; risotto; salmon with beurre blanc sauce on a puree of sweet potato; bok choy; and spelt pasta. Tom Van Asbroeck, another up-and-comer who posted several top-ten finishes in the 2014 racing season, ate all of these things as well as a few slices of bread with hazelnut butter. Nick van der Lijke, at twenty-three years of age the youngest member of the team, passed on the pasta and the bread and took his salmon without sauce. He did, however, enjoy a glass of wine, which is made available to the cyclists at every dinner.

Dessert was a new concoction from the bread lab of Frank van Eerd, a dense cake made with brown rice, plums, cherries, dark chocolate, and just a sprinkle of sugar. Van der Lijke ate two bites and pushed it away. I snarfed mine in two minutes and was tempted to ask van der Lijke for the rest of his.

Elite Endurance Athletes Eat Everything

The few days I spent with the LottoNL-Jumbo professional bike racing team revealed to me that its members practice all five habits of the Endurance Diet. Even Habit 5, eating individually, was on full display, despite the fact that the sixteen cyclists took all of their meals together. As you saw from the examples given in the previous section, no two plates were identical.

Habit 4, eating enough, was even more evident. Recall that this habit entails regulating food intake by paying mindful attention to internal signals of hunger and satiety. Unlike many restrained eaters, who often undereat, the LottoNL-Jumbo cyclists did not count calories or measure portions, and yet, unlike many mindless eaters who tend to overeat, these cyclists frequently left food on their plates.

Equally difficult to overlook was the cyclists' practice of Habit 3, eating carb-centered. The team's diet was jam-packed with carbohydrate-rich foods, from the crepe with apple butter that Maarten Wynants ate for breakfast to the lasagna and focaccia that Laurens ten Dam ate for lunch to the pasta and risotto that Tom Van Asbroeck ate with his dinner.

Habit 2, eating quality, was exhibited as well. Almost everything the team ate belonged to one of the six categories of high-quality foods (vegetables; fruits; nuts, seeds, and healthy oils; unprocessed meat and seafood; whole grains; and dairy). The only low-quality food types they consumed were refined grains and the occasional sweet. They ate no processed meats or fried foods whatsoever.

If I had to pick one Endurance Diet habit that team LottoNL-Jumbo best exemplified, however, it would be Habit 1: eating everything. The balance and variety in their diet were truly impressive. Few riders left their table in the Sala Oriente after any meal without having consumed all six high-quality food types, not to mention healthy beverages such as unsweetened coffee, tea, and wine.

Take another look at Sep Vanmarcke's lunch. The focaccia he ate checked the boxes for whole grains (spelt), dairy (cheese), and vegetables (olives, etc.). Granted, it contained only a small amount of vegetables; but the salad he ate with it was *all* vegetables except for the added pine nuts and dressing, both of which belong to the category of nuts, seeds, and healthy oils. The unprocessed meat category was covered by the turkey slices Vanmarcke selected, and the pineapple chunks he had for dessert took care of the last category, fruit. His dessert of yogurt added more dairy and the homemade energy bar he left with doubled up on the whole grain, fruits, and nuts, seeds, and healthy oils categories.

The riders not only ate a balance of all six high-quality food types but also consumed a wide range of foods within each category. Consider Frank van Eerd's baking, for example. Van Eerd works with no fewer than eighteen different grains (none of which is wheat or corn). His breads and other baked goods frequently contain a variety of nuts, seeds, and fruits as well.

Eating everything means eating some low-quality foods, too. Sweets and refined grains added to the variety of the LottoNL-Jumbo team's diet in Mojácar Playa. Although their meals and snacks were dominated by high-quality food types, nothing was explicitly forbidden or completely avoided. Recall that gummy candies were among the items available to them in the soigneurs' rooms.

The LottoNL-Jumbo professional bike racing team is not unusual in this way. Choose an elite endurance athlete at random and you are almost certain to discover that he or she eats everything. Take Gina Crawford, a professional triathlete from New Zealand who has won thirteen iron-distance events. Her typical breakfast is a homemade porridge with oats (whole grain), chia seeds (nuts, seeds, and healthy oils), flaxseed (same), coconut (fruit), raisins (same), and whole creamy organic milk (dairy), supplemented with seasonal fruit. Lunch is often boiled or scrambled eggs or an omelet (unprocessed meat and seafood) with seasonal vegetables or a tossed salad (vegetable), cheese (dairy) on toast (whole grain), and more fruit. Dinner is another balanced meal with chicken, beef, or venison (unprocessed meat and seafood), brown rice (whole grain) or potatoes (vegetable), and a big salad (vegetable). Dessert consists of yet more fruit plus yogurt (dairy) or ice cream (sweet).

Why You Should Eat Everything

There are three reasons why you should follow the example of the LottoNL-Jumbo cycling team, Gina Crawford, and other elites and eat everything. First, eating everything is healthy. Second, eating everything is natural. And third, eating everything is enjoyable.

Eating Everything Is Healthy

On January 26, 2012, London's *Daily Mail* newspaper published a story about a seventeen-year-old girl named Stacey Irvine, who had recently been rushed to the hospital after she collapsed at home with breathing difficulty. Tests done there revealed that she suffered from severe anemia, inflamed veins in her tongue, and multiple vitamin deficiencies, which were treated with vitamin injections. But what made this story newsworthy was *the reason* Stacey Irvine collapsed. The teen told doctors that she had subsisted on a diet of fast-food chicken nuggets since she was a toddler. She had never eaten a single fruit or vegetable that she could remember and the only food she ate regularly besides chicken nuggets was French fries. Her drink of choice was Coke.

Stacey Irvine's story is an extreme example of the consequences of eating a diet with too little variety. Sure, she could have picked a better food than chicken nuggets to eat three times a day, but she would have developed health problems on *any* single-food diet. Only one food in nature contains all of the nutrients required to support human life: breast milk. Everything else is incomplete. Even foods we think of as very healthy would eventually kill us if we ate them exclusively. Vegetables are certainly very healthy, but no vegetable contains all nine essential amino acids that the body needs to build the proteins we're made of. If you ate nothing else besides spinach you would die of heart failure at some point.

It is possible to live on just two foods, if you choose the right pair. But research has shown that people are healthiest when they eat a wide variety of foods. In 1987, Susan and James Krebs-Smith analyzed the diets of 3,701 American men, women, and children. A tool called the Mean Adequacy Ratio (MAR) was used to assess how well each subject's diet satisfied basic human nutritional needs. The Krebs-Smiths also collected information on how often the subjects ate foods of different types. When these two measurements—MAR and dietary variety—were compared, it was discovered that the subjects whose diet included the greatest variety in food types did the best job of meeting their nutritional needs.

Nearly twenty years later, Suzanne Murphy at the University of Hawaii went a step further, dividing each basic food type into subtypes and measuring how often each subtype was consumed by each of ten thousand adult subjects. Separately, Murphy quantified the subjects' intake of healthy nutrients such as vitamins and unhealthy nutrients such as refined sugar. She found that people who ate a wider variety of food types consumed more healthy nutrients and fewer unhealthy nutrients and that people who ate a wider variety of *sub*types consumed even more of the good stuff and even less of the bad stuff.

There is some evidence that the benefits of dietary variety extend beyond food types and subtypes to individual foods. A 2006 study involving Iranian women revealed that those who ate the greatest variety of whole grains were most likely to get enough vitamin B2, while those who ate the greatest variety of fruits were most likely to get enough vitamin C, and the women who ate the greatest variety of meats were most likely to get enough protein.

So it appears that dietary variety is beneficial at every level, from types to subtypes to specific foods. Variety at the level of basic food types is most important, though. Put another way, it is healthier to eat just one food of each of the six high-quality food types than it is to eat six different foods of any single type. The reason is that foods within each type are not as diverse nutritionally as are foods of different types.

Each high-quality food type has a distinct but limited nutrient profile that is complementary to the other types. Vegetables contain a more diverse array of antioxidants than fruits, which contain more fiber than nuts, seeds, and healthy oils, which contain more unsaturated fat than unprocessed meat and seafood, which contain more protein than whole grains, which contain more starch than dairy, which contains more probiotics than vegetables. A diet that includes a balance of all six of these food types is therefore more nutritionally complete than is a less inclusive diet.

Each high-quality food type supports health in a different way. The antioxidants in vegetables prevent cellular wear and tear, the fiber in fruit promotes digestive health, the fats in nuts, seeds, and healthy oils are good for the nervous system, the protein in unprocessed meat and seafood supports tissue regeneration, the starch in grains provides energy for both mental and physical exertion, and the probiotics in certain dairy foods benefit immune function. What's more, the health effects of the various high-quality food types are synergistic. Each food type is more beneficial when the other five are also included in the diet.

Before the 1980s, nutrition scientists tended to study the health effects of individual nutrients, foods, and food types in isolation. But over the past thirty years nutrition scientists have put greater emphasis on identifying the healthiest combination of food types. There is now a general consensus that a diet including all six high-quality food types is best. This consensus is based on a number of large-scale epidemiological studies including a 2014 study undertaken as part of the ambitious Dietary Patterns Methods Project. Its authors reported that, within a population of 424,000 older men and women, those who ate all of the high-quality food types most frequently were more than 20 percent less likely to die of heart disease, cancer, and other causes over a fifteen-year period compared to others.

Such findings have immediate relevance to endurance athletes and exercisers, because overall health is the foundation of endurance fitness. Every component of health is a component of endurance fitness also. Consider these few examples:

Antioxidant defenses: Nonathletes need strong antioxidant defenses to prevent bodily wear and tear and to slow the aging process. Endurance athletes need even stronger antioxidant defenses to absorb the stress of training.

Lean body composition: Nonathletes need a lean body composition to minimize their risk for a long list of chronic diseases. Endurance athletes need to be even leaner to maximize their efficiency of movement on the racecourse.

Insulin sensitivity: Nonathletes need their body tissues—particularly their muscles—to be highly sensitive to the action of the hormone insulin, so that they are better able to absorb and utilize carbohydrates obtained from food, leaving fewer carbs to be converted to body fat or get stuck in the bloodstream and wreak havoc. Endurance athletes need even greater insulin sensitivity to burn carbs effectively during workouts and races.

Each of the six high-quality food types makes a unique contribution to endurance fitness. Vegetables promote a lean body composition; fruit helps the immune system stand up to the stress of training; nuts, seeds, and healthy oils keep postworkout inflammation in check; unprocessed meat and seafood enables the muscles, bones, and connective tissues to adapt to training; grains provide fast fuel for workouts; and dairy accelerates muscle refueling and repair.

Eating Everything Is Natural

The story of humanity is largely a story of dietary diversification. Scientists believe that several million years ago our primate ancestors survived on a diet that consisted primarily of fruits, leaves, and insects. That's already a fairly diverse (technically omnivorous) diet, but our forebears were just getting started.

At some point—exactly when is not known—some of these proto-apes took a chance on living off the savannah, adding new foods such as grasses to their diet. Those who stayed behind in the trees continued to eat fruits, leaves, and insects, as chimpanzees (their direct descendants) still do today. This first genealogical split was followed by many others. At each fork in the road, it was the lineage that went down the path of greater omnivorousness that led a step closer to modern humans.

Slightly less than two million years ago, for example, a particular lineage known as hominins split into two groups. Analyses of food residues left in the fossilized teeth of each species indicate that *Paranthropus* had a relatively narrow diet based on grasses and sedges, whereas *Homo* had a broader diet that mixed grasses and sedges with foods from trees, shrubs, and herbs, as well as from the animals that ate these same foods. Guess who faded out and who became us?

Paleobiologists have proposed that one of the reasons why the primate, hominin, and human lineages that expanded their diet tended to outlast those that clung to narrow tradition was that a diverse diet offered greater security. The more omnivorous a species or subspecies was, the more options it had to fall back on when climatic or other environmental changes eliminated an important food source.

Such security comes at a cost, though. A species such as ours that is long accustomed to a highly varied diet becomes nutritionally *dependent* on dietary diversity. Because humans have such a long history of omnivorousness, we require a balanced and inclusive diet to sustain optimal health. A lion can live a long and vigorous life without ever eating anything but antelope meat. Poor Stacey Irvine showed us what happens when a person tries something similar.

Anatomically modern humans have existed for about two hundred thousand years. Roughly one hundred thousand years ago, our ancestors began to spread out from Africa to populate the planet. As they wandered, separate groups encountered many new foods, causing the overall diet of the species to become even more diverse. For example, a tribe known as the Ainu arrived on the island of Japan roughly fourteen thousand years ago and began to eat seaweed—not something their ancestors had eaten very much of.

Until recently, scientists knew little about the biological mechanisms that made such abrupt dietary shifts possible. It is now recognized that the microbiome, a collection of bacterial colonies that live in our gut and do much of our digestive work for us, are largely responsible. The microbiome is astonishingly adaptable, altering its composition and function on various timescales in response to dietary changes. Returning to the example just mentioned, the Ainu, through contact with marine microbes, quickly acquired microbiotic genes that produce enzymes that make seaweed more digestible.

By 10,000 BC, the nomadic era of human history had more or less come to an end. Individual populations settled down in their chosen environments, shifted from food gathering to food production, and gradually developed distinct cultural cuisines based on favored local foods. If the prior era of human history was characterized by increasing dietary diversity, this new age was a time of dietary winnowing. Each society domesticated select plants and animals and pretty much gave up eating everything else. Their diets remained diverse, though, because people still craved variety in their eating and human health still depended on variety, and a diverse food economy was still needed for food security.

What is most remarkable about the various cultural cuisines that developed in different parts of the world is their overarching similarity. Humans everywhere chose the same general types of foods to domesticate and incorporate into their cuisines. Populations from South America to Siberia based their diet on five food types: vegetables; fruits; nuts, seeds, and oils; meat and seafood; and grains; and a sixth food type, dairy, was added somewhat later in Europe, North Africa, the Indian Subcontinent, and a handful of other places.

The Maya, who thrived in Central America between 2000 BC and 250 BC, ate lots of squash and beans (vegetables), papaya and pineapple (fruits), Maya nuts (nuts, seeds, and healthy oils), turkey and shellfish (unprocessed meat and seafood), and corn (grain). The Assamese people of precolonial India were fond of yams and gourds (vegetables), bananas (fruit), betel nuts (nuts, seeds, and healthy oils), duck and sol fish (meat and seafood), rice (grain), and curds (dairy). Medieval Britons ate (among other things) carrots and cabbage (vegetables), plums and blackberries (fruit), hazelnuts and acorns (nuts, seeds, and healthy oils), mutton and herring (unprocessed meat and seafood), breads made from wheat, rye, and barley (grains), and cheese (dairy). You get the idea.

The next big change in human diet occurred in the age of industrialization, which began in the nineteenth century. This era witnessed the development and popularization of processed foods made from the five or six natural food types that all traditional cultural cuisines had been based on for centuries. Four particular types of processed foods became central to modern diets: refined grains, sweets, processed meats, and fried foods. Whole wheat bread was turned into Wonder Bread, milk into ice cream, pork into bologna, and potatoes into potato chips, as it were.

Unlike the natural whole foods they come from, these four types of processed foods are linked to negative health consequences such as obesity and heart disease. The explosive increase in the rates of diet-related chronic diseases that occurred in the last part of the twentieth century in particular gave rise to a general notion that the modern human diet was in a fallen state—that we had gone off track with our eating. Although the evidence clearly showed that it had happened in the industrial age with the propagation of the four types of low-quality processed foods, some people placed our fall much earlier. Proponents of the Paleo Diet argued that we never should have started eating grains, dairy, or even legumes, and that we should stop eating these foods now. Vegetarian diet advocates argued that we never should have started eating seafood, meat, and dairy, and should reverse those errors today.

Although they disagree on exactly when and how humans fell from dietary grace, all modern advocates of restricted diets agree that it is *unnatural* for humans to eat everything. However, an unbiased look at human history teaches us not only that it is natural for humans to eat everything, but that eating everything is what made us human in the first place and what continues to define us as human even now. When any species of animal, humans included, is coerced into defying its own nature, bad things happen. For this reason, I believe that endurance athletes (and anyone else seeking health and happiness) should include not only all six high-quality food types in their diet but the four low-category food types as well. I will say more about why you should allow yourself to eat refined grains, sweets, processed meats, and fried foods in the last section of this chapter.

Eating Everything Is Enjoyable

All animals like what is good for them. Evolution wouldn't work very well otherwise. The joy of sex apotheosizes the link between pleasure and survival. The same principle also applies to diet. Each species possesses a hardwired attraction to its natural food sources.

Humans not only are programmed to like certain flavors, such as sweet, but we also have a built-in liking for diversity in our foods. Evidence of this predilection comes from studies on the effect of food variety on energy intake. In one such study, six young men spent nine days in a clinical environment where they had free access to food, but the variety of offerings was manipulated. When the variety of the food was minimal, the men ate 15 percent fewer calories than they did when the number of options was maximal, presumably because they got bored with eating the same things. Scientists refer to this phenomenon as sensory-specific satiety.

In theory, it's possible that this preference for variety in the diet is learned—something society imposes on people—rather than genetically rooted. But research involving young children, whose eating choices are based more on instinct and less on acculturation, suggests otherwise. In a 2012 experiment, researchers at Cornell University and London Metropolitan University created images of forty-eight dinner plates featuring different combinations of foods and asked twenty-three children between the ages of five and twelve years to choose their favorite. The most diverse plates contained six foods, and those were the ones that a majority of the children selected. Adults presented with the same images favored plates with three foods. So it would appear that acculturation tends to narrow our naturally diverse food tastes rather than expand them.

The origins of this taste for eclecticism are ancient. As I mentioned above, even the common ancestor we share with chimpanzees was omnivorous, so it is not surprising that scientists have learned that modern monkeys also like to mix things up in their diet. In 2010, scientists at Duke University and the Institute of Cognitive Science and Technology in Rome taught capuchin monkeys to use tokens to barter for food. After identifying the monkeys' favorite food type, the researchers gave them the option to trade tokens for a large amount of that one type of food or for an assortment of foods that included their favorite as well as several others that they did not like as much. They went for the variety pack.

In a report published in *Behavioural Processes*, the experimenters wrote, "These results suggest that variety-seeking is rooted in our evolutionary history, and that it satisfies the need of experiencing stimulation from the environment; at the ultimate level, variety-seeking may allow the organism to exploit novel foods and obtain a correct nutritional intake."

This observation closes the loop on the three reasons endurance athletes (and humans in general) should eat everything. We enjoy eating everything because it is natural for us to eat everything, and it is natural for us to eat everything because it is healthy for us to eat everything.

The Costs of Not Eating Everything

Although nearly all elite endurance athletes eat everything, many recreational endurance athletes and exercisers do not, and when they don't, there's almost always a price to be paid. In some cases the costs are physical. In other cases the negative effects are mainly psychological but no less harmful to health, fitness, and performance.

Physical Consequences

In my experience, the three high-quality food types that are most often absent in the diets of recreational endurance athletes and exercisers are vegetables, unprocessed meat and seafood, and whole grains. I haven't yet encountered anyone whose diet lacked all of these food types. Rather, individual endurance fitness seekers tend to avoid just one of the three.

Athletes and exercisers (not to mention sedentary individuals) who avoid eating vegetables do so not because they think veggies are unhealthy but simply because they don't like them. These men and women typically eat some vegetables (and, no, potato chips don't count!), but not enough of them to escape physical consequences, which can range from poor recovery to increased risk for colds and flu.

An example is Brandon, a subelite runner from Ohio who was attempting to qualify for the US Olympic Trials Marathon when I worked with him. Brandon was raised on a particularly low-quality version of the Standard American Diet and stayed on it throughout college. He told me that he did not eat a single vegetable during his five years as an NCAA student athlete. His youth kept him out of trouble for a while, but eventually he began to suffer from fatigue, poor recovery, and recurrent injuries. A physician traced these problems to Brandon's adrenal glands, which play a key role in the body's response to all kinds of stress. His diet was so poor in key vitamins that his adrenal glands had become overtaxed, unable to manage the stress of his training. Brandon changed his diet and his problems went away.

Unlike veggie haters, athletes who shun meat and seafood do so intentionally, often but not always because they believe they will be healthier and perform better without animal foods in their diet. The problem I see with the greatest frequency in athletes on plant-based diets is iron-deficiency anemia. This problem is common even in omnivorous athletes, and it is possible to avoid it on a meatless diet, but it becomes that much more difficult to avoid when the most iron-rich foods (e.g., beef and shellfish) are excluded from the diet.

One of the many anemic vegetarians I've worked with is Claudia, who reached out to me in 2012 after unusual muscle pains and lethargy sent her to a sports medicine clinic, where testing revealed that she was severely anemic. Claudia was shocked by the diagnosis because she had been vegetarian for several years. But I see this quite often.

The removal of meat from the diet does not always lead directly to iron deficiency and anemia. In many cases it just leaves athletes more vulnerable to being pushed over the edge by some other factor, such as stress or increased training.

Many athletes do just fine on a vegetarian or vegan diet, but you never know how your body is going to react to the elimination of animal foods. Another athlete I've advised, a triathlete from Florida named Maria, placed herself on a carefully planned vegan diet for four months and then spent the next four years trying to recover from immune system and adrenal disruptions that virtually shut down her training and caused frequent and diverse illnesses.

Grain avoidance has become increasingly popular among endurance athletes and exercisers in recent years. In many instances this unnatural restriction leads to chronic fatigue, poor recovery, and other symptoms of overtraining syndrome, such as mood and sleep disturbances. An example is Julie, a runner from my home state of New Hampshire, who came to me after a disastrous foray into something called the No Sugar No Grains (NSNG) diet.

"I felt awful," she told me. "It didn't just slow me down—I could barely even run at all."

I asked Julie what sorts of problems she'd been experiencing on her normal diet that motivated her to try NSNG. Her answer? "None." Julie had just been talked into it by some friends who were already on the diet. These same friends urged her to stick with NSNG despite the sabotage it was wreaking upon her training, insisting that she would eventually "adapt." She did not adapt, and after several weeks she pulled the plug.

There are plenty of anecdotal reports of athletes who swear they are thriving on a grain-free diet. But I've counseled enough Julies to know that, if not impossible, it's a lot harder to absorb intensive training on a grain-free diet than it is on the Endurance Diet, just as it's harder but not impossible to avoid iron deficiency on a plant-based diet. My question is this: Why make it harder for yourself?

Psychological Consequences

Most advocates of unnaturally restrictive diets for endurance athletes completely ignore the psychology of food, but I believe it's just as important as the physical side. Indeed, I have never encountered an endurance athlete who was unhappy with his or her diet and happy with his or her training and racing. To experience lasting success as an athlete, you need more than a healthy diet. You must also be happy with your healthy diet—and diets that forbid entire food types breed unhappy eaters. More specifically, diets based on the total elimination of one or more high-quality food types promote a fear- and guilt-based relationship with food that takes the fun out of eating, creates stress around food, and in some cases leads to full-blown eating disorders.

Returning to the case of Julie and the No Sugar No Grain diet, not only did she feel lousy on it, but she also really missed eating sugar and grains. Eating wasn't as fun without her morning pumpkin muffin. Worse, the NSNG diet culture that she found herself immersed in had a distinctly negative ethos that brought her spirits down every time she interacted with it (not surprising for a diet whose name contains four words, two of which are "no").

"I was appalled by how people treated each other on their [online] forum," she told me.

It seemed to her that everyone was competing to be the purest and most loyal representative of the diet, and just waiting for an opportunity to pounce on someone who revealed himself or herself to be less than 100 percent committed. Julie felt as if she had woken up in some bizarre dietary police state. When she quit the diet she had to cut all ties with the culture in order to get her equanimity back.

The risk of psychological consequences is present even when low-quality food types alone are purged from the diet. From a purely physiological perspective, there is no reason not to completely do away with refined grains, sweets, processed meats, and fried foods. There are no health or performance benefits to be gained from eating these food types. Yet I recommend that endurance athletes include them in their diet nonetheless. There are three good reasons to do so.

First, eating refined grains, sweets, processed meats, and fried foods in small amounts does no harm. Proof of this claim is to be found in the fact that most elite endurance athletes enjoy them as occasional treats. (The riders on the LottoNL-Jumbo team, I was told, have a tradition of eating French fries on the final day of the Tour de France.) You can be sure that if eating small amounts of low-quality foods reduced performance by even one half of 1 percent, they would be wholly absent from the diets of all successful elite endurance athletes.

Second, many low-quality foods taste really good. That's the whole reason we created them in the first place! One may argue (I wouldn't) that it was a mistake to create them, but they exist now and are normal parts of diets all over the world. I strongly believe that foods that bring pleasure but not physical health have a place, albeit as small one, in the diets of all health-seeking persons, including competitive endurance athletes. Indeed, because pleasure itself is healthy, a diet that includes a modicum of pleasurable but unhealthy foods is better for overall mind-body health than a diet that excludes these delicious low-quality items.

Finally, total eradication of all low-quality foods from the diet fosters the same unwholesome relationship with food that diets like NSNG do and produces the same consequences. Remember Brandon, the Olympic Trials aspirant? After he cleaned up his diet, Brandon hired a sports nutritionist to help him continue the process. Unfortunately, he hired a sports nutritionist who forced rigid restrictions upon him, forbidding the consumption of any sweets, fried foods, or alcohol. And that was just the beginning. She prescribed precise calorie counts and (highly restrictive) carbohydrate amounts for every meal he ate and even told him exactly when he was required to eat. After a few weeks on this stifling regimen, Brandon felt that he was no longer eating food but math.

Overall, he was on board with the program. The new Brandon was more than willing to load up on the vegetables that he used to push away. But he developed a persistent fear of eating the wrong thing and was wracked with guilt whenever he broke a rule. These feelings intensified after Brandon ate sweet potato fries at a restaurant dinner with his wife and some friends and posted a photo of the meal on Facebook, which his nutritionist saw and later rebuked him for.

Brandon's next big race was the USA Half Marathon Championship. Although he had avoided injuries and his diet was immaculate, he felt terrible from the very start and dropped out before he reached the finish line. Upon returning home, he went on an extended junk food bender and gained 10 pounds.

This is an all-too-common scenario. Ironically, the person who is most likely to eat an entire box of cookies is not the one who eats a cookie every day but rather the one who tries to avoid ever eating a single cookie. In 2015, researchers at the University of Canterbury in New Zealand invited subjects to fill out a questionnaire that collected information about their psychological orientation toward food. The subjects were first asked to state whether they associated chocolate cake with "celebration" or "guilt." The researchers found that those who chose guilt "reported unhealthier eating habits and lower levels of perceived behavioural control over healthy eating when under stress . . . and did not have more positive attitudes towards healthy eating."

When I started to work with Brandon, I told him that developing a positive, healthy relationship with food was every bit as important as eating healthily. The most successful endurance athletes have what I call a "yes-saying" attitude toward their diet. They don't just eat healthily—they're also contented in their diet. Athletes whose relationship with food is based on fear and guilt always end up sabotaging their fitness and performance in one way or another, even though their diets look good "on paper" most of the time. I explained to Brandon that one of the most important steps toward developing a healthy relationship with food is to eat everything, a habit that is also best for endurance fitness on a purely physiological level.

It took some time, but Brandon eventually stopped worrying about his diet even as his nutritional standards remained high. "It's not only simplified my approach to eating," he told me by e-mail, "but it's reduced a ton of stress around wondering if I've made the right food options in the right amounts."

How to Eat Everything

Putting the first habit of the Endurance Diet into practice couldn't be simpler. Step one is to reintroduce to your diet any food types you currently avoid, unless you cannot eat them because of a food allergy or intolerance. Step two is to make sure you eat all six high-quality food types regularly. Vegetables and fruits should be included in almost every meal and snack. With the others—nuts, seeds, and healthy oils; unprocessed meat and seafood; whole grains; and dairy—there is more flexibility. Each of these food types should be consumed at least a few times every week and may be eaten as often as a few times a day. The Diet Quality Score, a tool that I will introduce in the next chapter, will guide you toward eating each of the high-quality food types with sufficient frequency and consuming low-quality foods in amounts that don't impede progress toward your goals.

4   Habit 2: Eat Quality

THE LEGENDARY BRAZILIAN TRIATHLETE FERNANDA KELLER FINISHED THIRD at the Ironman World Championship a record six times between 1994 and 2000. I met Keller at Ironman Brazil in 1998, when I was working as a staff editor for *Triathlete*. The job didn't pay very well but the travel perks more than made up for the small salary. My trip to the beautiful coastal city of Porto Seguro to report on the first Ironman ever staged in South America was just one of many memorable junkets I enjoyed during my time with the magazine.

Arriving two days before the race, I checked into a resort hotel where most of the foreign triathletes, including a number of Americans, were staying. I spent the next day exploring the area. As I wandered through Porto Seguro's bustling streets, I was struck by the predominance of restaurants serving familiar foods—especially pizza, sushi, and hamburgers. My assumption at the time was that these establishments catered to tourists, but I learned later that these foods are quite popular in Brazil. I was more interested, however, in sampling Bahian regional specialties such as moqueca (a stew of fish and coconut milk) and acarajé (a fried dough made with mashed peas), which were also widely obtainable.

On race morning, I got out of bed well before sunrise and made my way to the beach, where I found a surprisingly large crowd of spectators, about half of whom looked as though they had come straight from the dance clubs. As a national hero, Fernanda Keller drew enthusiastic cheers from these onlookers when she splashed out of the Atlantic Ocean in third place after completing the 2.4-mile swim. I hitched a ride on the back of a photographer's motorcycle to watch the 112-mile cycling leg. We left the city outskirts and soon entered a different world, a soupy jungle dotted here and there with squalid shacks. We were trailing American Ken Glah, the leader of the men's race, when he emptied the last sip of Gatorade from a plastic squeeze bottle into his mouth and dropped it to the road. A pack of scrawny, shirtless boys chased after the three-dollar trifle as it skittered away from Glah's $2,000 time-trial machine.

In the women's race, Keller passed Jan Wanklyn and Claudia di Silva during the cycling leg to move into the lead, but she was in turn passed by American Heather Fuhr, the defending Ironman world champion, halfway through the marathon and crossed the finish line as the runner-up. I found Keller a short time later in a VIP tent, where she lay prone on a massage table as her battered and depleted muscles were gently kneaded. I introduced myself and asked a few questions about the race, scribbling shorthand versions of her answers down on a moist notepad. Keller was exhausted and her English imperfect, but she managed to communicate her radiant positivity flawlessly, and her overflowing joie de vivre required no translation. It did not surprise me at all that when I contacted Keller seventeen years later in connection with this book, she was still competing in Ironman triathlons at age fifty-one.

Passion has been a major factor in Keller's longevity. ("I will never retire because I have an athlete's soul," she said in one interview.) But so has her diet. A physical education major at the University of Rio de Janeiro when she discovered triathlon in the early 1980s, Keller has always taken great care with her diet and has publicly advocated her approach to healthy eating with great gusto. At the time I met her, Keller was finalizing plans to launch the Fernanda Keller Institute. Based in her home city of Niterói (located just outside of Rio de Janeiro), the institute, which still exists, provides health services to underprivileged children who suffer from either malnutrition or obesity, as a majority of impoverished Brazilian boys and girls do. The kids participate in exercise classes (swimming, cycling, and running, of course), receive individual attention from a nutritionist, are fed healthy snacks, and even take field trips to a supermarket with their parents to learn how to make good food choices on a budget.

There is nothing complicated or surprising about the dietary philosophy that Keller advocates and practices at home. She focuses not on calories or on specific nutrients but rather on food types, filling up on what she calls *alimentos saudáveis* (healthy foods) and minimizing her intake of *alimentos não saudáveis* (unhealthy foods). These concepts of healthy and unhealthy line up almost exactly with the Endurance Diet concepts of high and low quality. Keller's healthy staples include vegetables, fruits and fruit juices, whole grains, olive oil, fish and poultry, and yogurt and cheese. The unhealthy foods she tries to eat least often are sweets and soft drinks, red meat, fried foods, and alcohol. But she does not martyr herself to these standards.

"I eat pasta, ice cream, chocolate," she said in a 2003 interview. They're not part of my athlete's diet, but I can eat everything . . . Just avoid exaggerations. I'm not that boring radical who does not put anything in her mouth."

At the height of her racing career, Keller's typical day started with a five o'clock wake-up. She ate a hearty breakfast of whole-grain toast with cheese, mashed banana with oats and honey, a homemade orange juice/strawberry/blueberry smoothie, and coffee with milk. After finishing her meal, she rode her bike. When that was done, she snacked on dried apricots and a granola bar. Lunch was another large meal, consisting of rice and beans, baked fish, grilled mixed vegetables (often potato, eggplant, and squash), and also a salad of lettuce, carrots, tomatoes, and chia seeds dressed with olive oil and sea salt. Following her afternoon workouts (a run, a swim, and perhaps also a weightlifting or yoga session), Keller ate another snack—this time a slice of carrot cake with goji berries and a cup of jasmine tea. Dinner was usually more fish alongside a salad of quinoa and vegetables and a cup of grape juice. She drank water, coconut water, and fresh-squeezed fruit juice throughout the day.

This diet was quite normal for elite Brazilian endurance athletes at the time of my 1998 visit to Porto Seguro, and it remains so today. I am assured of this by my friend Marina Bonilha, who works as a nutritionist at the Pinheiros Sports Club in São Paolo. Founded in 1899, Pinheiros is the training home to many of Brazil's top runners and swimmers, including Cesar Ciélo, winner of nineteen Olympic and world championships medals. A cafeteria inside the facility serves member athletes three meals a day. Bonilha generously translated my Elite Athlete Diet Questionnaire into Portuguese and distributed it to several of the competitors she worked with. Among them were Adriana Aparecida da Silva, a 2:32 marathoner; Guilherme Guido, a swimmer who has represented Brazil in several world championships; Valdilene dos Santos, who has a personal best time of 16:21 for 5000 meters; and Joanna Maranhão, a three-time Olympian in swimming.

When I analyzed the completed questionnaires, I was not surprised to find that they contained many of Fernanda Keller's *alimentos saudáveis* and not a lot of the Endurance Diet's four low-quality food types. Maranhão stated that her preferred breakfast was tapioca with one egg and one egg white, cottage cheese, and turkey breast; a small plate of fruits (papaya, avocado, and strawberry) with chia seeds, flaxseed, and a bit of honey; and black coffee. Brown rice and beans were present on the lunch plates of most of the athletes, including that of dos Santos, who ate this modified Brazilian staple (white rice being the norm among nonathletes) with chicken or beef, a green salad, and either fruit or gelatin for dessert. The athletes' snacks were equally high quality. Da Silva's favorite consisted of yogurt with fruit, a rice cake, and coffee with milk. For most of them, dinner added further variety to the day's menu. A typical dinner for Guido was baked fish, sweet potato, and salad.

Brazilian elite endurance athletes are not alone in maintaining very high quality standards in their diet. Nearly all of the professional racers whose diets I have examined eat a lot of high-quality foods and few low-quality foods.

What Is Diet Quality?

Simply put, a high-quality diet is a healthy diet. When nutrition scientists talk about "high-quality" and "low-quality" foods, they mean the same thing that nonscientists like Fernanda Keller mean when they talk about "healthy" and "unhealthy" foods.

Scientists rate the quality of foods in a straightforward way: by studying their effects on human health. This is done principally through epidemiological studies, where information about the diets of hundreds or thousands of people is matched against disease rates within the same population. In particular, scientists look for associations between the frequency with which certain foods are eaten and the risk for obesity, type 2 diabetes, and cardiovascular disease, the three most pervasive diet-related health problems. Other diseases and conditions that have dietary links and can be used in the scientific assessment of diet quality are high blood pressure, Alzheimer's disease, unfavorable cholesterol levels, certain types of cancer, and systemic inflammation.

The limitation of this type of research is that it is not able to definitively prove causation. The fact that heavy coffee drinkers have a lower-than-normal risk for depression, for example, does not prove that coffee prevents depression. It's possible (though highly improbable) that some genetic factor that attracts people to coffee also protects against this disease. However, when an association between a certain type of food and a particular disease keeps appearing again and again in epidemiological studies, there is good reason to suspect a causal link. As the expression goes, "Where there's smoke, there's fire." Most of the evidence that smoking causes lung cancer comes from epidemiological research, after all.

In order to strengthen causal links suggested by nutritional epidemiology, scientists often follow up this type of research with interventional studies. In these studies, the food type in question is either added to or subtracted from the diets of volunteers for a period of time while their health is tracked. The limitation of this type of research is that, for ethical reasons, scientists cannot change people's diets in ways that are expected to harm their health; they can only test changes that are expected to be beneficial.

There is an important distinction to be made between a high-quality *food* and a high-quality *diet*. Like food quality, diet quality is judged by health outcomes. But diets are more complex and trickier to define than are individual foods. Common sense suggests that the healthiest (i.e., highest quality) diets will include a balance of most or all of the individual food types that are known to positively affect health and only small amounts of the foods that increase disease risk. But what is the optimal balance and how do we identify it?

In tackling this question it can be helpful to flip the usual approach to epidemiological research on its head. Instead of learning what people eat and then finding out how their food choices impact their health, researchers can seek out a group of exceptionally healthy people and learn what they eat. This is the approach that scientists have taken to studying so-called blue zones—areas where people tend to be unusually long lived. Diet is not the only factor that contributes to exceptional longevity in these places, but there is a consistent diet pattern in all of them. Specifically, people living in blue zones typically eat a balance of all six high-quality food types, with emphasis on plant foods, and only small amounts of the low-quality food types.

An example is Sardinia, an island off the coast of Italy where people are up to twenty times more likely to live beyond their 100th birthday than are people in the United States. The foods that Sardinians eat most often include beans and artichokes (vegetables), figs and grapes (fruit), almonds and olive oil (nuts, seeds, and healthy oils), barley (whole grain), and sheep's milk cheese (dairy). Meats and seafood—mainly lamb and shellfish—are typically eaten only once or twice a week but are a regular feature of the diet. White bread is the most commonly eaten low-quality food type. Sweets, processed meats, and fried foods have little place in the traditional Sardinian diet.

A high-quality diet benefits endurance athletes and exercisers in three ways. For starters, it increases overall health, and as I've mentioned already, general health is the foundation of endurance fitness. But each high-quality food type also contributes to endurance fitness in direct ways. I will specify these contributions later in the chapter. Finally, a high-quality diet helps endurance athletes and exercisers by being nutritionally efficient. People who engage in vigorous cardio exercise need to get as much overall nutrition as possible from each calorie in their diet. Doing so allows them to meet their general nutritional needs, which are elevated by training, without gaining or retaining excess body fat. Raising the overall quality of the diet enables endurance fitness seekers to meet their body's total nutritional needs without compromising body composition and achieve a leaner body composition without failing to meet the body's total nutritional needs.

The Diet Quality Score

The Diet Quality Score (DQS) is a tool that I developed a number of years ago to make it easy for athletes to monitor and improve their diet quality. The DQS assigns to each food type a point value that reflects its quality in relation to other food types. These point values serve to encourage users to sustain high diet quality in the same way elite endurance athletes and long-lived blue zone inhabitants do: by eating a balance of all six high-quality food types frequently and the four low-quality food types less frequently.

But here's the twist: These point values are not necessarily fixed. There is a tendency for the value of each food type to decrease based on how many times it has already been eaten in a given day. For example, the first and second servings of whole grains eaten in a day earn 2 points each, the third serving earns 1 point, the fourth and fifth earn 0 points, and the sixth subtracts a point from the day's DQS. This pattern reflects the fact that even the healthiest food types offer diminishing returns when eaten in abundance, and incentivizes users of the tool to eat a variety of food types.

To generate a Diet Quality Score, all you have to do is track how often you eat each type of food over the course of a day and assign the appropriate point value to each eating occasion. At the end of the day, after you've eaten your last food and added its point value to your tally, you will have your DQS for that day. I can assure you that this process is far less onerous than counting calories, and my DQS smart phone app (available in iPhone and Droid versions) makes it even easier.

The trickiest part of using the DQS is deciding what constitutes a scorable occasion of eating a given food type. These decisions start with knowing your food types. For example, is orange juice a fruit or something else? Complete definitions of each food type are given below. In addition to the six types of high-quality foods and the four types of low-quality foods, there are four "catch-all" categories for foods that don't fit within the basic types. These are "high-quality processed foods" (yes, they do exist), "high-quality beverages," "low-quality beverages," and "other."

Many foods are composites of two or more types. An example is my wife's homemade gumbo, which contains a roux (a heavy broth); tomatoes, peppers, and onions; crab and shrimp; Andouille sausage; and chicken wings. I encourage DQS users to exercise common sense in scoring such foods. In this example, I score the roux as "other" (the category for all heavy sauces, condiments, and gravies), the tomatoes, peppers, and onions as a half serving of vegetables (because they are included in relatively small amounts), the crab and shrimp as unprocessed meat and seafood, the sausage as a processed meat, and the chicken wings as a fried food.

I receive lots of e-mails from athletes who want to know how they should score a certain food that defies easy categorization. (It's telling that there are so many of them in the modern diet.) I am always happy to share what I think, but I also invite them to disagree with my judgment and come to their own decision. Although I did create the Diet Quality Score, I have no wish to be the final judge of how every food on Earth is classified for scoring purposes. This tool will work best for you if you can take some ownership of it and confidently make your own judgments when they are called for. It will become second-nature and more intuitive as you use the DQS.

Of course, it's not only *what* you've eaten but also *how much* that you must consider when defining occasions of eating particular food types. Returning to an earlier example, orange juice may be scored either as a half serving of fruit or as a high-quality beverage—either way it's valued at 1 point. But how much orange juice do you have to drink to earn that point? And how much more do you have to drink before it should be counted as two servings? In place of official serving sizes, which often fail to reflect the amounts of food that people actually eat, I counsel DQS users to define their own serving sizes based on what is normal for them. In other words, a serving is, for DQS purposes, the amount of a given food you normally eat. A larger man with a heavy training load and a hearty appetite might not be satisfied with less than a cup of (precooked) oats in his morning porridge and should therefore count that amount as one serving of whole grains, whereas a smaller woman with a lighter exercise regimen and a smaller appetite might only need a half cup (the "official" serving size) to achieve satiety and should count *that* amount as one serving for her.

Serving sizes can also be somewhat flexible even for each individual. For example, if I eat a slice of toasted whole-wheat bread with fruit spread at breakfast, I count it as one serving of whole grain. And if I eat two slices of the same bread in a sandwich, I also count it as one serving of whole grain. This allowance may seem wildly permissive, but the Diet Quality Score is not a tool that aims for scientific precision; it aims to be helpful to fitness-seeking individuals, and I have found that the use of flexible serving sizes renders the tool easier to use than it would be with official serving sizes and does not result in any significant loss of accuracy as a measure of diet quality.

This does not mean that *any* amount of a given food you consume should be counted as one serving, however. If you eat a single jelly bean, don't count it as a serving—or even a half serving—of sweets. Nor should you credit one grape as a serving (or half serving) of fruit. If you put two or more kinds of fruit in a smoothie, go ahead and count that as two servings. A few grilled peppers and onions stuffed inside an omelet should probably be counted as a half serving of vegetables. I think you get the idea.

These guidelines were not found inscribed on stone tablets and brought down from a mountaintop. I developed them on the basis of my judgment and experience. For judging portion sizes, most DQS users develop their own systems, which differ—not significantly, but slightly—from other peoples' systems. As long as the standards you apply are consistent, the tool will serve its purpose of accurately assessing your diet quality and allowing for methodical improvement. If you prefer a little more hand-holding initially, look to the "typical serving sizes" given in the next section and to the DQS counts given with Georgie Fear's recipes in Chapter 11.

If you are already familiar with the DQS, you may notice in reading the next section that the point values of some food types have changed slightly. These minor adjustments reflect knowledge I've gained from epidemiological research that has been done since the previous iteration of the DQS was released and from my ongoing study of elite athlete diets.

Below you will find tables with scoring rules for all of the DQS food types, as well as additional scoring guidelines and information about which specific foods are included within each category. The food types are presented in descending order of quality, an order that is based on how often elite endurance athletes eat them and is influenced by research on the effects of the various food types on the risk for, and treatment of, overweight, type 2 diabetes, cardiovascular disease, and, to a lesser extent, other diseases and conditions related to diet quality. The highest-ranked food types have the strongest positive health effects and are most beneficial when eaten frequently. These same foods also make the greatest positive contributions to endurance fitness. The lowest-ranked foods have the strongest negative health effects and must be eaten infrequently (though not eschewed completely) if these effects are to be avoided.

High-Quality Food Types

Vegetables; fruits; nuts, seeds, and healthy oils; whole grains; dairy foods; and unprocessed meat and seafood add points to your daily DQS.

Vegetables

Serving	1	2	3	4	5	6
Points	+2	+2	+2	+1	0	0

Vegetables are, alongside fruits, the highest-quality foods. They support general health and endurance fitness more effectively than any other single food type. Dozens of studies have demonstrated that the people who eat the most vegetables have the lowest risk for developing common chronic diseases, are the least likely to become overweight, and are the healthiest in old age. For example, a 2011 study involving more than 134,000 Chinese adults found that men and women who ate the most vegetables were 16 percent less likely to die over a ten-year period than those who ate the least vegetables.

The healthful effects of vegetables are attributed to their high concentration of fiber, vitamins, minerals, and antioxidants. Recent research has revealed that certain toxins in vegetables that give them a bitter flavor are also responsible for their health benefits. In living plants, these toxins protect against pests. But, in the human body, they provoke a mild stress response that leads to health-increasing physiological adaptations—just as exercise itself does.

In addition to helping the cells of the body resist aging, the antioxidants in vegetables protect them from oxidative stress during exercise, a cause of muscle damage and fatigue. In a 2005 study, researchers at the University of Newcastle investigated the effects of reduced vegetable and fruit intake in endurance athletes. Two weeks on this diet increased markers of oxidative stress after an exhaustive workout by 45 percent. A vegetable- and fruit-restricted diet also increased perceived effort during the workout—in other words, it made exercise feel harder.

Other research has shown that the health benefits of vegetable and fruit consumption plateau at five combined servings per day. This is why the DQS point value of both food types drops from +2 to +1 at four servings and from +1 to 0 at five servings.

Scoring Guidelines for Vegetables

The vegetable category includes whole fresh vegetables eaten raw
   or cooked as well as canned and frozen vegetables and pureed or
   liquefied vegetables used in soups, sauces, and so forth. Legumes

(peas, lentils, etc.) are also counted as vegetables in the DQS. Typical serving sizes of vegetables include a fist-size portion of solid vegetables, one-half cup of tomato sauce, and a medium-size bowl of vegetable soup or salad.

One hundred percent vegetable juices may be counted either as one-half vegetable serving or as high-quality beverages.

Fruits that are generally regarded as vegetables for culinary purposes—including tomatoes and avocados—may be counted as vegetables.

A composite food containing more than one type of vegetable may be counted as one-and-a-half or two servings of vegetables. But don't automatically count such foods as multiple servings. Consider the overall size of the food portion. For example, don't count a side salad of greens, cucumbers, and carrots as three vegetable servings just because it contains three different vegetables. Count it as one serving.

A little iceberg lettuce and a thin pink tomato slice on a hamburger should not be counted as even one-half portion of vegetables. Generous amounts of vegetables on a sandwich may be counted as one-half portion of vegetables.

Vegetable-based Foods

Nonfried vegetable snack chips such as kale chips should be counted as high-quality processed foods unless they contain added oils, in which case they should be counted as fried food even if they are not fried.

Plant-based powder supplements such as Greens Plus should be counted as high-quality processed foods, not as vegetables.

Soy products such as soy burgers and other processed foods made entirely or almost entirely from vegetables should be counted as high-quality processed foods.

Spinach pasta and spinach tortillas should not be scored as vegetables. They should be counted as refined grains unless made with whole grain.

When in doubt about whether to count a particular processed or composite food as a vegetable, don't. Instead count it as a high-quality processed food.

Fruit

Serving	1	2	3	4	5	6
Points	+2	+2	+2	+1	0	0

Fruit carries the same health and fitness benefits as vegetables, for the simple reason that fruits are nutritionally very similar to vegetables. Like vegetables, fruits are rich in fiber, vitamins, minerals, and antioxidants. One significant difference between fruit and vegetables is that the carbs in fruit are mostly sugar, whereas those in vegetables are mostly starch. Lately, concerns about the health effects of sugar have motivated many health-conscious people to limit their fruit intake, but these fears are completely unfounded. Whereas processed foods and beverages containing added sugars have been linked to weight gain and other undesirable outcomes, fruit has not.

In fact, fruit *prevents* weight gain and facilitates weight loss more effectively than almost any other food type. In a scientific review published in 2009, Danish researchers looked at past research on the relationship between fruit intake and body weight. Of sixteen studies analyzed, eleven showed that elevated fruit intake either prevented weight gain or induced weight loss.

Scoring Guidelines for Fruit

The fruit category includes whole fresh fruits, canned and frozen fruits, cooked whole fruits, blended fruits, dried fruits, and foods made with whole fruits such as apple sauce. Typical serving sizes of fruit include one medium-size piece of whole fruit (e.g., one banana), a handful of berries, and one-half cup of apple sauce.

Foods that include multiple fruits, such as smoothies, may be counted as one-and-a-half to two servings of fruit.

Fruit-based Foods

Small amounts of fruit included in baked goods, packaged yogurt, etc., should not be counted.

One hundred percent fruit juice may be counted either as a half serving of fruit or as a high-quality beverage. Juice products that are less than 100 percent fruit juice and contain added sugars should be counted as sweets.

Fruit-based desserts such as peach cobbler may be double-scored as fruits and sweets.

Fruit-based products such as dried cranberries and applesauce that contain added sugar should be double-scored as fruits and sweets.

All processed fruit snacks such as Fruit Roll-Ups should be counted as sweets.

Fruits such as tomatoes and avocados that are treated as vegetables in culinary tradition may be counted as vegetables.

Nuts, Seeds, and Healthy Oils

Serving	1	2	3	4	5	6
Points	+2	+2	+1	0	0	-1

Nuts, seeds, and natural oils extracted from these foods and from other whole plant foods such as olives are rich in unsaturated fats and plant sterols that promote favorable blood cholesterol profiles and healthy arteries.

The health effects of nut consumption in particular have been widely studied. Frequent nut eaters are less likely to die of type 2 diabetes, respiratory disease, heart disease, and certain types of cancer. They also have lower levels of body fat than do people who eat nuts less often. According to a 2014 review by scientists at Purdue University, nuts promote a lean body composition because they are highly satiating, they displace lower-quality foods from the diet, the calories in them are not absorbed efficiently by the body, and perhaps also because they increase metabolism and fat burning.

The health benefits of seeds and oils (other than olive oil, which I'll discuss in greater detail in Chapter 10) have not been studied as thoroughly as those of nuts, but what research has been done so far indicates these benefits are equivalent to those of nuts. Animal studies have demonstrated, for example, that olive oil boosts the body's ability to defend itself against free radical damage to muscle fibers during endurance exercise.

Because nuts are so filling, it's best not to eat them quite as often as you eat vegetables and fruits, lest they start to displace other high-quality foods from your diet. For this reason, their DQS point value drops earlier and more steeply than do those of vegetables and fruits.

Scoring Guidelines for Nuts, Seeds, and Healthy Oils

The nuts, seeds, and healthy oils category includes cashews, almonds, walnuts, sunflower seeds, hempseeds, flaxseeds, chia seeds, and other such foods. Peanuts should be counted as nuts although they are technically legumes. Typical serving sizes in this category include a palmful of nuts or seeds, enough peanut butter to cover a slice of bread, and two tablespoons of salad dressing.

This category also includes non-chemically extracted plant oils consumed raw or cooked in small amounts. For example, an olive oil– or flaxseed oil–based dressing on a salad is to be counted as a serving of healthy oil, as is grape seed oil or avocado oil used to sauté vegetables.

Nut and seed butters made without sugar or other additives besides salt should be counted as nuts, seeds, and healthy oils. Those made with added sugar should be counted as sweets.

Baking flours made from *whole* nuts or seeds, such as Bob's Red Mill Super-Fine Almond Flour, count as nuts, seeds, and healthy oils.

Heavily coated or candied nut- or seed-based foods such as glazed peanuts, peanut brittle, and chocolate-covered almonds should be counted as sweets.

Whole Grains

Serving	1	2	3	4	5	6
Points	+2	+2	+1	0	0	-1

According to the theories that support low-carb diets, whole grains *ought* to have negative effects on body weight, type 2 diabetes, and cardiovascular disease because of their high carbohydrate content. But a veritable avalanche of research indicates that men and women who eat whole grains frequently are leaner, are less likely to develop type 2 diabetes and cardiovascular disease, and even live longer than those who eat them infrequently.

In addition to preventing weight gain and the chronic diseases associated with it, whole grains help reverse such conditions in those who already have them.

The beneficial effects of whole grains on the risk for chronic diseases appears to be mediated in part by the food's tendency to reduce systemic inflammation, which is an underlying factor in many such conditions.

Like vegetables and fruits, whole grains owe their beneficial health effects to their combination of fiber, vitamins, minerals, and antioxidants. The greatest difference between whole grains and vegetables and fruits is that whole grains are more energy dense. For example, one-half cup of brown rice supplies 108 calories, 90 of them from carbohydrates. One-half cup of peas supplies only 62 calories, 46 of them from carbs. The high carbohydrate density of whole grains makes them terrific fuel for endurance training. It also makes them easier to overeat than vegetables and fruits are. This is why the maximum number of DQS points achievable in one day from whole-grain intake is 5, or 2 points fewer than vegetables and fruits offer.

Scoring Guidelines for Whole Grains

The whole-grain category includes whole wheat, buckwheat, barley, brown rice, corn, oats, amaranth, quinoa, spelt, bulgur, millet, rye, sorghum, and teff. It also includes breads and other baked goods, pastas, breakfast cereals, and other grain-based foods made with 100 percent whole grains and no refined grains.

Whole-bean flours such as garbanzo bean flour should be counted as whole grains even though, technically, they are processed legumes.

Homemade popcorn counts as a whole grain. (Movie theater popcorn, microwave popcorn, and bagged, ready-to-eat popcorn do not.)

Typical serving sizes of whole grains include two slices of bread, a medium-size bowl of breakfast cereal, and a fist-size portion of brown rice, quinoa, etc.

Dairy

Serving	1	2	3	4	5	6
Points	+2	+1	+1	0	-1	-2

Not that long ago, dairy was widely considered to be a low-quality food except in low-fat versions. But recent science has shown that the fats in dairy products are a key source of their health benefits. In a 2015 study, Swedish researchers found that the risk for type 2 diabetes was lower among men and women who frequently consumed full-fat dairy products and slightly higher in those who often consumed low-fat dairy products. Whole milk and foods made from it also promote healthy cholesterol profiles and improve vascular function.

All forms of full-fat dairy have positive health effects except for butter (and clarified butter or ghee). Although butter is harmless when included in the diet in small amounts, people who use a lot of butter exhibit less favorable cholesterol profiles. New research suggests that the reason has to do with butter's lack of a membrane enclosing fat molecules that is present in other forms of dairy.

Fermented dairy products, yogurt especially, confer additional health benefits through their impact on gut bacteria. There is evidence that these foods lower blood pressure, offer relief for certain digestive disorders, reduce systemic inflammation, reduce breast cancer risk, prevent weight gain, and facilitate the loss of excess body fat.

A little dairy goes a long way, though. Its benefits are maximized at just one or two servings per day. And because dairy is energy dense, consuming it in large amounts may present challenges for weight management. In the DQS, the point value of dairy turns negative after the fourth serving of the day to discourage overconsumption.

Of note to endurance athletes and exercisers, the two main proteins in milk—whey and casein—have been shown in studies to prevent muscle damage during exercise and accelerate muscle recovery after workouts.

Scoring Guidelines for Dairy

The dairy category includes whole cow's milk, goat's milk, sheep's milk, all cheeses, yogurt, sour cream, kefir, cream cheese, and cottage cheese.

Eaten in small amounts (e.g., a thin pat spread on toast), butter, clarified butter, and ghee should not be scored. Eaten in larger amounts (e.g., lobster dipped in melted butter), they should be counted as a heavy sauce and scored in the "Other" category.

Low-fat milk, skim milk, and all other reduced-fat dairy foods are counted as half servings of dairy because they are not as beneficial as their whole counterparts.

Dairy-based Foods

All sweetened dairy products, including ice cream, frozen yogurt, sweet cream, chocolate milk, and yogurts containing some form of sugar as their second ingredient should be counted as sweets.

Nondairy milk and cheese products made with high-quality foods (soy milk, rice milk, tofu cheese, etc.) should be counted as high-quality processed foods.

Typical serving sizes of dairy include the amount of milk you would normally use in a bowl of breakfast cereal, two slices of deli cheese, and a single-serving tub of yogurt.

Unprocessed Meat and Seafood

Serving	1	2	3	4	5	6
Points	+2	+1	+1	+0	-1	-2

Research on the health effects of eating seafood has consistently shown that it reduces the risk of cardiovascular disease by enhancing vascular function, lowering blood pressure, and reducing systemic inflammation. Seafood is also good for the brain and nervous system. Some studies have reported that regular fish eaters exhibit better brain function in old age and are less likely to become depressed or to develop Alzheimer's disease. All of these benefits are attributed primarily to the omega-3 fats in seafood.

Seafood and the omega-3 fats in it offers endurance-specific benefits as well. In 2014, Polish researchers reported that three weeks of supplementation with omega-3 fats increased production of nitric oxide (which causes blood vessels to dilate, increasing blood flow during exercise) and elevated VO_2max in elite cyclists.

Research on the health effects of meat is more mixed. Studies have generally found that white meat neither improves nor impairs health. Some investigators have reported that high red meat intake increases the risk for cardiovascular disease and reduces life span. And there is a definite association between red meat and elevated risk for colorectal cancer. But a large epidemiological study performed recently by Swiss researchers found that only processed red meat was linked to negative health outcomes and that people who ate small amounts of unprocessed meat lived longer than vegetarians.

All in all, it seems most prudent to consume unprocessed meat and seafood in modest amounts. The DQS point value of this category is set to encourage such moderation. Within the category, I recommend eating seafood more often than white meat and white meat more often than red meat.

Scoring Guidelines for Unprocessed Meat and Seafood
The unprocessed meat and seafood category includes unprocessed
skeletal and organ meats from all commonly eaten land animals

as well as the flesh of all commonly eaten sea animals. See the
subsection on processed meat for a definition of "processed."

Eggs of all types (chicken, duck, etc.) should be counted as
unprocessed meat and seafood.

Canned, jarred, and frozen meat and seafood products count as
unprocessed only if they do not contain significant amounts of
low-quality food ingredients. For example, pickled herring, which
typically contains vinegar, a bit of sugar, and spices, can be scored
as unprocessed meat and seafood.

Typical serving sizes in this category include one chicken breast, a
hand-size filet of fish, and two eggs.

Low-Quality Food Types

Refined grains; sweets; processed meat; and fried foods subtract points
from your daily DQS.

Refined Grains

Serving	1	2	3	4	5	6
Points	-1	-1	-2	-2	-2	-2

Refined grains are whole grains that have been stripped of some of their
best parts. Through this process, they also lose health benefits, including their favorable effect on body composition. In 2010, scientists at
Tufts University reported that, within a population of 2,843 men and
women, higher intake of whole grains was associated with lower body
fat levels, but just the opposite was true of high refined-grain intakes.

Although less healthy than whole grains, refined grains remain a
good source of carbohydrate fuel for training and recovery. It is perhaps
for this reason that refined grains are the most commonly consumed
low-quality food type among elite endurance athletes. Many elite Japanese athletes, for example, prefer white rice to brown rice. This would
not be the case if refined grains were as detrimental to health and
fitness as the other three low-quality food types. Indeed, although the

USDA cautions Americans to consume sweets "sparingly," the agency's MyPlate guidelines permit up to half of the grains in the diet to come from refined sources.

I encourage endurance athletes to aim higher, however, as elite racers in most parts of the world now do. By assigning a negative point value to even the first serving of refined grain consumed on a given day, the DQS incentivizes you to choose whole grains whenever possible, except for occasions when you want a special treat.

Scoring Guidelines for Refined Grains

The refined grains category includes white rice, processed flours, and all breakfast cereals, pastas, breads, and other baked goods made with less than 100 percent whole grains.

Note that, in wheat-containing products, any description other than "whole wheat," "whole wheat flour," or "whole grain wheat flour" indicates that the wheat is refined and the product should be counted as a refined grain.

Breakfast cereals containing more than 10 grams of sugar per serving should be counted as sweets, unless they contain dried fruit.

Whole-grain baked goods should be counted as sweets if they contain enough sugar to taste sweet.

Typical serving sizes of refined grains include a fist-size portion of white rice, a medium-size bowl of pasta or breakfast cereal, and two slices of bread.

Sweets

Serving	1	2	3	4	5	6
Points	-2	-2	-2	-2	-2	-2

There's no denying the fact that foods and beverages containing refined sugar are unhealthy. A 2014 study reported that men and women who got more than 25 percent of their calories from added sugar were more than twice as likely to die of cardiovascular disease over an eighteen-year period compared to those who got less than 10 percent of their calories from added sugar. (The diet of the average American is 13 percent added sugar.)

Added sugar is everywhere in our food supply these days. It takes a consistent effort to avoid it, in part because it is disguised under so many names (look out for barley malt, brown rice syrup, cane syrup, corn syrup, dextrose, high-fructose corn syrup, and sucrose). The DQS incentivizes the avoidance effort by assigning a point value of -2 to each serving of sweets.

Scoring Guidelines for Sweets

The sweets category includes all foods and beverages containing substantial amounts of refined sugars, including candy, pastries, and other desserts.

Sugary drinks may be scored either as low-quality beverages or as sweets (the point values are the same).

All foods sweetened artificially should be counted as sweets. Artificially sweetened beverages should be counted as low-quality beverages.

Energy bars and snack bars not made with whole grains, fruit, and/or nuts should be counted as sweets unless consumed during exercise, in which case they should not be scored.

Breakfast cereals with more than 10 grams of sugar per serving are to be considered sweets unless they contain dried fruit.

All fruit juices containing added sugar and all processed fruit snacks such as Fruit Roll-Ups should be counted as sweets.

Yogurt products containing some form of sugar as their second ingredient should be counted as sweets.

Agave nectar is marketed as a natural food but is in fact highly processed. It should be counted as a sweet.

Sweets Counted as Other Foods

Honey and maple syrup are not counted as sweets unless used in large amounts. Although high in sugar, they are natural whole foods that have been a part of the human diet for eons.

Dark chocolate does not count as a sweet (don't score it at all) if it's
at least 70 percent cacao and consumed in small amounts
(100 calories or fewer).

Typical serving sizes of sweets include a slice of pie, a small candy bar,
and a 12-ounce can of soda.

Processed Meat

Serving	1	2	3	4	5	6
Points	-2	-2	-2	-2	-2	-2

Processed meats such as bacon are among the unhealthiest foods you
can eat. In small amounts they're harmless, but a large body of research
has shown that the heaviest eaters of processed meats face increased
risk for obesity, cardiovascular disease, type 2 diabetes, some cancers,
and early death. Scientists are still trying to pin down the mechanisms
involved. In the meantime, we know enough about processed meat to
assign it a fixed Diet Quality Score of -2 points.

Scoring Guidelines for Processed Meat

The processed meat category includes most forms of meat that have
been processed beyond basic cutting, grinding, and seasoning. It
encompasses sausages and other encased meats, most cold cuts,
jerky, bacon, other smoked meats, cured meats, corned beef, meat
loaf, hot dogs, chicken nuggets, and all fast-food meats except
high-quality exceptions such as whole chicken pieces and the
Carl's Jr. All-Natural Burger.

Charred and blackened meats should be counted as processed because
the charring and blackening processes create carcinogens.

Animal fats used for cooking, including bacon grease and lard, should
be counted as low-quality meats.

Typical serving sizes of processed meat include one hamburger patty,
three deli slices, and a two slices of bacon.

Fried Foods

Serving	1	2	3	4	5	6
Points	-2	-2	-2	-2	-2	-2

The frying process transforms even the healthiest foods into unhealthy foods by drastically increasing their energy density and introducing toxic compounds such as aldehydes. Take potatoes, for example. Boiled and baked potatoes are very healthful. A study published in the *Journal of the American College of Nutrition* reported that people lost weight after adding five to seven servings per week of nonfried potatoes to their diet. But according to a study by researchers at the Harvard School of Public Health, potato chips are responsible for more long-term weight gain in the United States than any other single food. It's best to reserve such foods for special treats.

Scoring Guidelines for Fried Foods

The fried foods category includes all deep-fried foods such as potato chips, fried chicken, fritters, and donuts.

All snack chips containing added oils should be counted as fried foods even if they are not actually fried (e.g., baked kale chips) because they are just as energy dense and addictive as their fried cousins.

Nonfried "Fried" Foods

Pan-fried, stir-fried, and sautéed foods do not count as fried foods.

Typical serving sizes of fried foods include a small bag of potato chips and one whole donut.

Additional Categories

Not all foods and beverages fit neatly into the ten categories I've just described. These additional categories are intended to fill the gaps.

Other

Serving	1	2	3	4	5	6
Points	-1	-2	-2	-2	-2	-2

This category includes the following:

- All condiments, sauces, dressings, and gravies except those that are made from high-quality whole foods, such as guacamole, hummus, mustard, pesto, and salsa (full servings of which may be scored as a half serving of the food type they belong to; obviously, typical serving sizes vary widely by the specific food—I suggest cueing off label or recipe guidelines)
- All calorie-containing nutritional supplements including protein powders and meal replacements except those made entirely from high-quality foods, such as vegetable powders
- Any food or beverage you come across that does not easily fit into any of the main food types

High-Quality Processed Foods

Serving	1	2	3	4	5	6
Points	+1	0	-1	-2	-2	-2

This category includes all processed foods made *entirely or almost entirely* from high-quality food sources. Examples are:

- Nondairy milk and cheese products (soy milk, rice milk, tofu cheese, etc.)
- Vegetarian alternatives to meat products made from high-quality food sources, such as all-vegetable veggie burgers
- Energy bars and snack bars made only from high-quality foods such as whole grains, nuts, seeds, and dried fruit
- Supplements made from high-quality food sources such as unsweetened whey protein powder
- "Diet" foods made from high-quality foods such as Quaker Weight Control Instant Oatmeal

High-Quality Beverages

Serving	1	2	3	4	5	6
Points	+1	+1	0	0	-1	-2

This category includes the following:

- The first alcoholic beverage consumed on a given day
- 100 percent fruit juice (which may also be scored as a half serving of fruit)
- 100 percent vegetable juice (which may also be scored as a half serving of vegetables)
- Blends of 100 percent fruit and vegetable juices
- Unsweetened and lightly sweetened coffee and tea

Milk should be counted as dairy. Nondairy milks (e.g., soy milk) should be counted as high-quality processed foods.

Typical serving sizes of high-quality beverages include an 8- to 12-ounce glass of fruit juice and a 6-ounce glass of wine.

Low-Quality Beverages

Serving	1	2	3	4	5	6
Points	-2	-2	-2	-2	-2	-2

This category includes the following:

- Sugary drinks (if not counted as sweets)
- Coffee drinks such as lattes containing more than 50 calories
- Artificially sweetened beverages
- Alcoholic beverages *after* the first of the day
- Sports drinks if consumed outside of exercise

Typical serving sizes of low-quality beverages include a 12-ounce can of diet soda and a 16-ounce latte.

The DQS in Action

We've established the DQS basics and guidelines; here's a snapshot of the DQS tool in practice. Reviewing it will help you use the same tool with greater confidence to assess the quality of your own diet.

Raiza Goulão is a Brazilian professional mountain biker with a very high-quality diet. But it's also a somewhat complex diet, which is why I chose it for this illustration. Table 4.1 presents a typical day's eating for her and shows how to generate a DQS from the information.

Table 4.1 An Elite Endurance Athlete's Diet Quality Score

Meals and Snacks	Remarks	DQS Points
Breakfast Homemade muesli with oats, quinoa, mixed dried fruits, flaxseed, chia seeds, and chestnuts; fruit juice	Given their variety, the muesli, quinoa, and oats may be counted as two servings of whole grain (+4); likewise, the flaxseed, chia seeds, and chestnuts may be scored as two servings of nuts, seeds, and healthy oils (+4); the mixed dried fruits are best counted as one-half serving of fruit (+1), as is the fruit juice (+1)	+10
Snack Fresh mango and papaya chunks	I'd count this snack as one serving of fruit (don't automatically count combinations of two foods of the same type as one-and-a-half or two servings unless the total amount is substantial)	+2
Lunch Grilled chicken; grilled mixed vegetables; salad with lettuce, diced tomato, grated apple, cheese, carrot oil, mint, grated ginger, banana slices, pineapple chunks, chestnuts, and capers	The grilled chicken represents one serving of unprocessed meat and seafood (+2); the grilled vegetables are one serving of vegetables (+2); the salad is one serving of vegetables (+2), one serving of fruit (+2), and one-half serving of nuts (+0.5 because it's the third serving of the day)	+9
Snack Smoothie with papaya, passion fruit, unflavored gelatin, mint, and brown sugar	Raiza Goulão has a sweet tooth. She manages it by eating lots of fruit and by putting small amounts sugar in otherwise high-quality foods like this smoothie. Normally, I score all foods with tasteable amounts of added sugar as sweets, but in this case I feel Goulão should not be penalized because she is making a good faith effort to minimize refined sugar consumption, and the amount of sugar used in the recipe is small. So I would score this snack as two servings of fruit (+3 because they're the third and fourth servings of the day) and 1 sweet (-2)	+1

(Continued)

Table 4.1   *Continued*

Meals and Snacks	Remarks	DQS Points
Dinner Crepes filled with shredded chicken, mixed cheeses, and tomatoes	The crepes, made with tapioca flour, are one serving of refined grain (-1); the shredded chicken is one serving of unprocessed meat and seafood (+1 because it's the second serving of the day); the cheeses are one serving of dairy (+2); the tomatoes are one-half vegetable serving (+1)	+3
Dessert Homemade dessert bread with rice flour, quinoa, chia seeds, flaxseeds, and yogurt, and 100 percent fruit preserves	The rice flour is one-half serving of refined grain (-1); the quinoa is one-half serving of whole grain (+0.5 because it's the third serving of the day); the chia seeds and flaxseeds are one serving of nuts (+0.5); the yogurt is one-half serving of dairy; the fruit preserves are one-half serving of fruit (+0.5)	+0.5
	Total:	24.5

How to Increase Your Diet Quality

The maximum DQS score for a day is 35 points. It is seldom if ever necessary to hit this mark to achieve health and fitness goals. Elite endurance athletes typically attain scores in the low to mid-20s. This level of diet quality seems to be "good enough" for them. Further increases in diet quality bring no additional benefits.

There is no single target Diet Quality Score that is right for everyone, however. The DQS score that is optimal for one person may not be optimal for another. Larger individuals and people who exercise a lot need to eat more than smaller and less active persons. This gives them more opportunities to add points to their DQS. So the optimal DQS for larger and more active men and women is typically higher.

Instead of aiming for a perfect or one-size-fits-all Diet Quality Score, I recommend that you make incremental improvements to your diet quality until you reach a point where you are happy with the health, fitness, and performance results you're getting but you're still enjoying what you eat (and still allowing yourself to eat small amounts of the low-quality foods you like). If you're the kind of person who absolutely *must* have some kind of target to aim for when using such a tool, start with a target of 20 points. But be open to adjusting this number based on what you learn from using the tool.

Tracking your DQS can be beneficial even without a target. The simple act of monitoring the quality of your diet will encourage you to make healthier choices. Most people think their diet is healthier than it actually is. In a survey by *Consumer Reports*, more than 90 percent of respondents rated their current diet as "healthy." Yet only 11 percent of Americans eat the government recommended five combined servings of fruits and vegetables per day. Clearly, there's a disconnect between subjective perceptions of diet quality and objective reality. When you track your DQS, you will no longer be able to kid yourself about how often you really eat high-quality and low-quality foods.

There are three ways to improve your diet quality. You can remove low-quality foods from your diet, you can add high-quality foods to your diet, and you can substitute low-quality foods with high-quality foods. Generally, I don't recommend removing low-quality foods from the diet without replacing them with high-quality alternatives because it is psychologically difficult to do. Low-quality beverages such as soda are an exception. The only acceptable alternative to these is water.

Substituting low-quality foods with high-quality foods works especially well because it can make a big difference in diet quality without feeling especially disruptive. The typical fast-food hamburger, for example, comes in at -4 to -6 points (depending on what the person eating it has already consumed that day). But if you prepare your own burger at home, you can replace the restaurant's low-quality beef (-2) with high-quality beef (+2), replace the white-flour bun (-1) with a whole wheat bun (+2), and replace the mayonnaise (-1) with guacamole and suddenly you've got yourself +4 points. You can gain an additional point by loading up your burger with enough veggies in addition to the guacamole (which should not be scored on its own if used in a small amount) to count as a half serving of vegetables—an example of adding high-quality foods to the diet.

If you are calorie conscious, you may fear that *adding* any foods— even high-quality foods—to your diet is a recipe for weight gain. But high-quality foods are highly satiating, so, when you add them to meals and snacks, you will tend to eat less later. In a sense, then, adding high-quality foods to your diet is really another form of substitution because it displaces other (lower-quality) foods, even if you're not aware of it.

Table 4.2 presents a few examples of the almost infinite variety of ways to improve Diet Quality Scores, especially via the methods of adding high-quality foods and substituting low-quality foods with high-quality foods. Other ways of improving diet quality are suggested in Chapter 10, where I present twenty-two "endurance superfoods"

Table 4.2   Some Ways to Improve Your Diet Quality

Method	Examples
Remove low-quality foods	Drink one serving less of soda per day
Add high-quality foods	Add vegetables (e.g., grilled peppers) to a breakfast omelet
	Add nuts and no-added-sugar dried fruit to oatmeal
	Turn a morning bagel into a bagel sandwich with veggies (see page 214)
	Drink vegetable juice with lunch
	Add vegetables (e.g., spinach) to fruit smoothies
	Use vegetables (e.g., tomatoes and olives) as pizza toppings
Substitute low-quality foods with high-quality foods	Replace café latte with lightly sweetened coffee
	Replace high-sugar, refined-grain breakfast cereal with low-sugar, whole-grain breakfast cereal and add fruit
	Replace refined-grain bread with 100 percent whole-grain bread in sandwiches
	Eat dinner leftovers instead of a sandwich for lunch
	Replace snack chips with mixed nuts
	Replace ham with turkey
	Replace postmeal cookie with one small piece of dark chocolate

that are popular among elite athletes and are among the first high-quality foods you should add to your diet if you're not already eating them. Replacing some of your current meal choices with the recipes shared in Chapter 11 will also help you raise your Diet Quality Score.

Once you have raised your diet quality to a level that brings you the results you seek, the hard work is over, and it is no longer necessary to track your Diet Quality Score daily. If you eat more or less the same types of meals and snacks each day, and if you've already scored them in the past, there is no need to score them again. The DQS tool is intended for use in changing your diet. When your new habits are locked in, use it only periodically to audit your diet for the sake of ensuring you're not unwittingly backsliding, to identify the potential cause of unexpected weight gain, and to maintain your standards when you travel and in other circumstances where your normal routine is disrupted.

The Other Quality

As I mentioned earlier, when scientists talk about quality in relation to diet, they're talking about the healthfulness of the diet. But when everyday people talk about quality in relation to diet, they are usually talking about the *grade* or *caliber* of a given food. For example, a filet mignon from a grass-fed cow might be called a high-quality cut of meat, while a hunk of ground chuck from an industrially raised cow might be labeled low quality.

There is overlap between "quality" in the scientific sense of healthy and "quality" in the colloquial sense of high grade. Spinach grown in healthy, nutrient-rich soil is likely to have a 20 to 30 percent greater vitamin and mineral content than regular supermarket spinach. Einkorn wheat, an ancient variety of the grain, is richer in unsaturated fat, zinc, iron, and several antioxidants than modern, industrial wheat varieties. Grass-fed beef has more conjugated linoleic acid and omega-3 fat and less saturated fat and total fat than grain-fed beef. Wild Alaskan salmon contains more omega-3s and less mercury than nonorganic farmed Atlantic salmon.

A diet that is high quality in both senses of the term is best for health and fitness. To maximize the quality of your diet in the scientific sense, you need only base your diet on the six high-quality food types. To maximize the quality of your diet in the popular sense, you need to select your high-quality foods carefully, buying locally grown, sustainably farmed fruits and vegetables sprouted from native or heritage seeds (and/or growing your own); wild seafood bearing the Marine Stewardship Council's Certified Sustainable Seafood Label; meat from free-range, grass-fed, and hormone- and antibiotic-free animals; organic dairy products and free-range eggs; and locally grown everything whenever possible.

The downside of pursuing this type of quality is that it can be expensive and less convenient than buying whatever the nearest supermarket carries. If the cost or hassle is too great for you, don't lose sleep over it. Raising your Diet Quality Score will do more for your health and fitness than switching to higher-grade foods of the same types you're already eating. Bear in mind that none of the research I've cited on the health benefits of vegetables; fruits; nuts, seeds, and healthy oils; whole grains; dairy; and unprocessed meat and seafood discriminated between high-grade and low-grade forms of these foods. Some apples may be better than other apples, but there are no bad apples.

5   Habit 3: Eat Carb-Centered

Vincent Onywera is a professor of exercise physiology at Kenyatta University, located just outside the Kenyan capital of Nairobi. His office on the fourth floor of the main administrative building is large and well appointed, befitting his stature as one of the school's most prominent faculty members. I met him there on a Monday afternoon in June of 2015. We settled into a couple of padded leather chairs facing each other across a low table and Onywera served tea, which he, like most Kenyans, drinks with plenty of milk and sugar.

Eleven years before this meeting, Onywera, then an exercise science graduate student at Kenyatta, made a name for himself by leading the first rigorous study of the diet of elite Kenyan runners. He and three colleagues spent a full week recording and measuring everything that went into the mouths of ten male athletes, including several world champions, at a high-altitude training camp in Eldoret, a hub of Kenya's elite running community. Onywera and his collaborators reported their findings in the *International Journal of Sport Nutrition and Exercise Metabolism*.

"The staple foods were bread, boiled rice, boiled potatoes, porridge, cabbage, kidney beans and *ugali* (a thick maize meal paste)," they noted. "Meat (mainly beef) was served at the training camp 4 times per week and consumed in modest amounts (approximately 100 g per day) although athletes were able to access more meat and other foods when visiting their rural homes. A significant amount of tea (with milk) was also consumed during the day."

Nearly all of the foods on this list of staples—which are common in the diet of Kenyan nonrunners as well—are high in carbohydrates. So it came as no surprise to Onywera's team to discover that the runners got more than 76 percent of their daily calories from carbs. (The average American's diet, by contrast, is about 48 percent carbohydrates.) Interestingly, all ten athletes lost body fat during the study period.

Kenya's runners are, as you probably know, the best in the world. Kenyan men account for a staggering seventeen of the twenty fastest male marathon times in history, while Kenyan women own fifteen of the twenty best female half-marathon performances of all time. I asked Onywera if he believed that the high carbohydrate content of the elite Kenyan runner's diet constituted an advantage with respect to runners from other nations. Onywera said it probably was an advantage. After all, their average daily carb intake of 10.4 grams per kilogram of body weight was consistent with the amounts that had been shown to maximize endurance performance in controlled studies and was somewhat greater than the amounts in the diets of athletes from most other countries.

Having jotted down this answer in my notebook, I then inquired whether Onywera was aware that a number of endurance sports nutrition gurus in the United States and elsewhere argued that low-carb diets were best for fitness and performance. He told me he was.

"So, what would happen," I asked, "if one of these gurus went to a training camp for elite Kenyan runners and told them their diet was all wrong—that they needed to go low-carb?"

"They would laugh," Onywera said, laughing himself. "They wouldn't take him seriously."

One week after my meeting with Vincent Onywera, I rented a room at the High Altitude Training Centre (HATC) in Iten, a village located just up the road from the Eldoret-based training camp whose athletes Onywera had studied. Created by retired runner and former half-marathon world record holder Lornah Kiplagat, HATC provides accommodations and facilities to a clientele made up primarily of foreign athletes who wish to spend a month or two training at high altitude with the world's best runners. I was there not to train, however, but to see for myself how top Kenyan runners eat.

Attached to the HATC is a club that serves somewhat more upscale food than the simple but high-quality fare provided in the Centre's dining room. On my second night in Iten, I shared a meal there with Timothy Limo, an elite 800-meter runner who provided coaching services for the HATC. He ordered fish stew with chapati (a kind of tortilla) and sukuma wiki (stewed collard greens). I asked for the same. While we ate, Limo described a typical day's eating for him and the runners he trained with.

"Our first run is very early, so we don't eat anything before it except maybe honey with water," he said.

(Interestingly, recent science has demonstrated a special benefit of doing some workouts in a fasted state—particularly a carb-fasted state—showing it causes a type of metabolic stress that enhances certain fitness adaptations. I will discuss carb-fasted workouts—which Kenyan runners do for pragmatic rather than scientific reasons—in Chapter 9.)

"After the run," Limo continued, "we drink chai [another name for Kenyan-style tea] and eat chapati or bread and bananas."

The runners give the food a little time to digest and then run again. "After the second run we eat uji," Limo said. "You know uji?" I did. It's a porridge made from fermented millet and often flavored with lemon juice. I'd eaten some earlier in my visit to Kenya and found it to be quite delicious.

Lunch, Limo continued, consists of rice or potatoes and githeri, a mixture of boiled maize and beans. At midafternoon, following the third run of the day or perhaps a core workout or massage, the runners eat another helping of uji. Dinner is most often ugali with meat or fish, sukumi wiki, and mursik (fermented milk).

I asked Limo if he and his training partners did much snacking. "Yes," he said. "We eat fruit—pineapple, mango, oranges, beetroot—anytime; whenever we're hungry."

Like the list of foods given in Vincent Onywera's landmark study, the foods Limo named in his review of his (and the typical Kenyan runner's) daily menu are almost all high in carbohydrates, starting with the honey taken early in the morning and culminating in the ugali that supplies a plurality of dinner calories. The only exceptions are the bit of meat or fish eaten at dinner (but not every night) and the beans and greens consumed frequently at lunch and dinner, which, although not high in carbohydrates, still contain more carbs than protein or fat.

Having confirmed that, more than a decade after Onywera completed his study, Kenyan runners still eat a lot of carbohydrates, I paid a visit on the following day to a nearby hotel owned by Wilson Kipsang, who until the previous year had held the world record in the marathon, to find out if the country's wealthiest and most widely traveled runners continue to eat traditional Kenyan cuisine or abandon it for "Western" alternatives.

Kipsang received me in his office—decorated with such noteworthy items of memorabilia as a mounted right shoe (the one in which he ran 2:03:23 at the 2013 Berlin Marathon) and a photograph taken of him with Prince Harry after winning the 2012 London Marathon—and promptly set about serving us tea. I asked him directly whether money (he took home more than $700,000 from his 2014 New York City Marathon victory alone) had changed the way he ate.

"I still eat the same foods," he said with a sly smile. "They're just more . . . accessible."

"What about when you travel to England or Germany or America to race?" I asked. "Do you eat their food or do you take ugali with you?" (I had heard of other Kenyan runners carrying bags of ugali on airplanes.)

"I eat their food," he said. "It's not a problem. I'm only there for a few days and I find other ways to get carbohydrates. Instead of ugali, I eat spaghetti."

Remembering my conversation with Vincent Onywera, I asked Kipsang if he was aware that many people in America and other wealthy nations say that carbohydrates are bad and should be avoided by runners and nonrunners alike. Just as the professor had predicted, he laughed.

"Why do they say that?" asked Kipsang, genuinely perplexed. "Carbohydrate is not bad!"

Carbohydrates, Fitness, and Performance

Although Kenya's elite runners are an extreme case, they are not the only elite endurance athletes who maintain a carbohydrate-centered diet. A 2011 study at the University of Potsdam found that elite junior triathletes from Germany consumed 9 grams of carbohydrate per kilogram of body weight daily during a period of intense training, only 13 percent less than the amount consumed by the Kenyan runners studied by Onywera.

In my research, I have found that virtually all elite endurance athletes on every continent put high-carbohydrate foods at the center of each meal and most snacks. If you select a world-class endurance athlete at random and analyze his or her diet, you are almost certain to find that he or she maintains a high level of carbohydrate intake.

A typical case is Radka Vodickova, a professional triathlete from the Czech Republic. Vodickova starts most days with a bowl of oatmeal with dried fruit and yogurt and a mug of green tea. She snacks on bananas, dried fruit, yogurt, and nuts. One of her go-to lunch menus is risotto with vegetables. Dinner is carbohydrate-centered as well, often consisting of chicken with rice or beef and potatoes accompanied by a nice big salad.

As much carbohydrate as most elite runners eat, however, Kenyan runners eat more. The many foreign athletes who stay at Lornah Kiplagat's High Altitude Training Centre, therefore, must adapt to an even higher level of carb intake than they are used to. The results are consistently positive. Among the runners whose stay at the HATC overlapped with mine were Yannick Michiels, a Belgian runner and orienteer who had run 13:47 for 5000 meters; Emmett Dunleavy, a 3:47 1500-meter runner who has represented Ireland at the world cross country championships; Anuradha Cooray, who holds Sri Lanka's national record in the marathon (2:13:47); and Elvan Abeleygesse, who holds Turkish national records at six distances. All of these athletes assured me that they responded quite well to the high-carb Kenyan diet. Both Dunleavy and Michiels had lost weight since arriving

at the Centre. Cooray told me that he'd lowered his marathon time by
two minutes after each of his three prior visits to Iten.

My own experience was similar. I ate traditional Kenyan foods
almost exclusively during the two weeks I spent in Kenya. Midway
through the trip, I ran the Safaricom Lewa Marathon, known as one
of the toughest marathons in the world because it takes place in hot
weather on a hilly off-road course at high elevation. I felt strong the
whole way and finished the race in seventeenth place overall, third
among runners over forty, and first among non-Kenyans. My body
recovered from the race with surprising speed. After two days off I was
back to running and feeling great.

A carbohydrate-centered diet offers several benefits to endurance
athletes and exercisers. For starters, it enables the body to better handle the stress of training. Any given training program will cause less
physiological stress—in the forms of muscle damage, inflammation,
immune system disruption, hormonal disturbances, and nervous system perturbations—on a diet that supplies adequate carbohydrates.
A 2015 study by researchers at the University of Western Australia,
for example, revealed that consecutive days of high-intensity training
caused significantly more inflammation in well-trained endurance athletes on a low-carb diet than on a high-carb diet.

Limiting the physiological stress of training is not just beneficial
for its own sake. It also enables athletes to gain fitness faster and perform better. This was shown in a 2004 study by Asker Jeukendrup and
colleagues at the University of Birmingham. Seven well-trained runners spent eleven days on each of two diets: a high-carb diet (8.5 grams
of carbohydrate per kilogram of body weight per day, or 65 percent of
total calories) and a low-carb diet (5.4 grams of carbs per kilogram per
day, or 41 percent of total calories). Their training load was increased
substantially for the last week of each eleven-day period. Before and
after this intensified training period, the runners completed a 16-kilo-
meter time trial. Performance in the time trial decreased significantly
after intensified training on the low-carb diet, but on the high-carb

diet performance held steady, indicating that the extra carbs enabled the runners' bodies to better absorb the hard work.

Because a carb-centered diet limits the physiological stress of training, switching to a low-carb diet is one of the riskiest things an elite endurance athlete can do nutritionally. It doesn't happen often, and, when it does, the results can be disastrous. The American mountain biker Georgia Gould offers one such cautionary tale. In 2010, Gould won her third national championship in the cross country discipline. The following year, she read a book whose author argued that carbohydrates are the primary cause of weight gain and type 2 diabetes. Gould found the argument persuasive and decided to adopt the high-fat, low-carb diet the book recommend. She greatly increased her meat consumption and virtually eliminated all grains from her meals.

Gould missed her next period. And the one after that. And the one after that. Ignoring the warning sign, she persisted with the new diet even though she hated it from the start. An avid cook, Gould no longer enjoyed being in the kitchen, feeling restricted by the inflexible rules of her low-carb eating plan. When she traveled, which was often, she worried about food constantly. Initially, she felt just a little off emotionally—not quite herself—but after several weeks she was teetering on the brink of a full-blown depression.

Midway through the 2011 racing season, the bottom fell out from under Gould's training and racing. She felt terrible on every training ride and produced the worst competitive results of her entire career. Only then did she see a doctor, who ran blood tests and discovered several abnormal hormone values and ordered her to change her diet. Gould went back on a high-carb diet, immediately recovered, and won the 2011 USA National Cross Country Mountain Bike Championship.

Going low-carb isn't quite as risky for recreational endurance athletes who train less than the pros, but the results of doing so are often decidedly negative for them, too. A typical case is Matthew Laye, an ultrarunner and university professor from Boise, Idaho. In 2014, Laye adopted a ketogenic diet, one of the most extreme low-carb diets, which requires its adherents to get at least 70 percent of their daily calories from fat and no more than 10 percent from carbohydrates. He expected to feel lousy initially as his body adapted to the new regimen, and he did. The problem was that he never stopped feeling lousy.

Even though a hamstring injury limited him to half of his normal training volume at this time, every workout was an ordeal. "I was running a minute per mile slower at the same level of effort in my easy runs," he told me, "and my ability to do any high-intensity work was severely compromised."

Other recreational endurance athletes who switch to a low-carb diet—and even the extreme ketogenic diet—report good results. However, I have not yet encountered any athlete who, when pressed, was able to point to a quantifiable breakthrough in performance after making such a change. At best, low-carb athletes get back to the same level they were at on their previous diet, and only after going through a long and often unpleasant period of adaptation. The "good results" they report have nothing to do with performance but instead consist of things like modest weight loss, improved digestion, and reduced reliance on sports drinks during longer races.

In a certain respect, low-carb diets are like veganism and other extreme diets that recreational endurance athletes choose. Although it is not impossible, at least for some people, to achieve a high level of fitness on such diets, it is certainly harder, and as I've asked before: Why make things harder for yourself?

And there are other negatives to consider beyond the possibility of feeling awful and performing poorly in training. Low-carb diets, and, in particular, high-fat, low-carb diets, are highly restrictive and culturally abnormal. The list of foods that are 70 percent fat or more is quite short. Athletes who try to get 70 percent of their total calories from fat often end up eating the same few foods—many of them low quality—over and over. When Matthew Laye went ketogenic he quickly discovered that in order to hit the 70 percent fat target he had to limit himself to a very small variety of foods. Fruits and grains were out of the question because it was impossible to compensate for their high carbohydrate and low fat content. He had to choose fatty processed meats such as bacon and salami over lean unprocessed meats such as chicken and turkey. His salads were drenched in oil and devoid of higher-carb ingredients such as carrots. "It was incredibly monotonous," he told me. "Even if the diet had worked for me, it would have been unsustainable for that reason alone."

Very low-carb diets are also nutritionally unbalanced. For example, the best food sources of magnesium—whole grains and beans—are often eliminated on such diets, resulting in magnesium deficiency and its consequences, which include muscle cramps. Another common health consequence of extreme carbohydrate restriction is unfavorable changes in blood lipids. Six weeks into his high-fat, low-carb diet, Laye got a cholesterol test and learned that his LDL ("bad") cholesterol level had jumped to 200 milligrams per deciliter, an increase of 39 milligrams per deciliter from before he went ketogenic. Soon afterward, he reverted to his old way of eating.

Additional, sometimes strange, health problems have been reported by low-carb eaters after they've been on the diet for a long time. Among these are vertigo, skin problems, panic attacks, and caffeine intolerance. Some of these issues may be related to stress placed on the liver by prolonged carbohydrate deprivation.

Finally, like other extreme diets, low-carb diets all-too-frequently function as a gateway to eating disorders. Studies indicate that a majority of cases of eating disorders are preceded by some form of dieting. Not all people who try a low-carb diet develop an eating disorder and not all people who develop an eating disorder use a low-carb or other extreme diet as a gateway, but the risk is one more reason to avoid them.

Yet another benefit of a carbohydrate-centered diet, beyond increased training capacity, greater fitness gains, and improved training performance, is better performance in competition. In 2009, Trent Stellingwerff of the Canadian Sports Centre in Victoria tracked the diets of 257 runners during the final five weeks before the London Marathon. Of these runners, thirty-one consumed 7 grams of carbs per kilogram of body weight or more before the race. The others ate less, and in many cases a lot less. The thirty-one runners who ate the most carbs completed the marathon 13.4 percent faster than a group of runners matched for gender, age, body weight, training volume, and marathon experience who ate less carbohydrate before the race. Most of this difference came in the final 4.5 miles, where the runners who had eaten fewer carbs hit the wall and slowed down precipitously.

Inadequate carbohydrate consumption not only reduces performance in longer races but also reduces aerobic capacity, or VO_2max, which is the most important element of endurance fitness. This was shown in a 2014 study published in the journal *Nutrients*. Polish researchers placed eight mountain bikers on each of two diets for four weeks in random order. One diet was high in fat and low in carbohydrates (HFLC), consisting of 15 percent carbohydrates, 70 percent fat, and 15 percent protein. The other diet was more balanced, consisting of 50 percent carbohydrates, 30 percent fat, and 20 percent protein. At the end of each dietary intervention, the participants were subjected to three days of physiological testing that culminated in a 90-minute stationary bike ride at 85 percent of lactate threshold power followed by a 15-minute time trial.

On average, the athletes' VO_2max was 2 percent higher after four weeks on the normal diet than it was after an equal amount of time on the high-fat, low-carb diet. This might not sound like much, but small differences in aerobic capacity translate to crucial differences in endurance performance. Indeed, the subjects were able to sustain an additional 12 watts in a 15-minute trial and 4 watts at lactate threshold intensity on a normal diet compared to a HFLC diet.

The rationale for going low-carb as an endurance athlete is that it trains the muscles to burn more fat and less carbohydrate during workouts and races. And it works. The mountain bikers included in the study just described burned fat at much higher rates during exercise after a month of high-fat, low-carb eating. But as the same study showed, better fat burning does not translate to better performance. In fact, the fittest and fastest endurance athletes are more often those who are able to burn carbohydrates, not fat, at the highest rate. A 2014 experiment led by Giuseppe Lippi and colleagues at the University of Verona found that levels of alpha-amylase—an enzyme that serves as a marker for carbohydrate-burning capacity—strongly predicted half-marathon performance in a group of forty-three recreational runners.

In light of this science, it's not at all surprising that almost all of the world's best endurance athletes practice Habit 3 of the Endurance Diet. But do they really? Advocates of low-carb diets often point out that some of the top ultrarunners in the world are on low-carb diets. The problem with these counterexamples is that, although ultrarunning is growing quickly in popularity and performance standards are on the rise, the sport has not yet reached the point where it is attracting the most talented athletes. For this reason, it is still possible for athletes with superior talent to win in the sport despite using inferior methods of preparation in diet and training, just as was the case in other endurance disciplines in past decades. I am confident that when ultrarunning does reach the point where it is as competitive as those other disciplines are today, the most successful athletes will be on carbohydrate-centered diets. Indeed, they will probably be Kenyan.

Carbophobia

According to a 2014 Gallup survey, 29 percent of Americans try to avoid eating carbohydrates. This statistic reflects a negative public attitude toward carbs that has been trending steadily upward since Gallup initiated its annual Consumption Habits Survey in 2003. In 2005, physician and author Michael Greger gave the phenomenon a name: *carbophobia*.

The main source of carbophobia is a seemingly endless series of popular low-carbohydrate diets developed outside the mainstream of nutrition science. These include the Atkins Diet, the South Beach Diet, and the Paleo Diet. Although such diets differ in their particulars, their creators share a common belief that carbohydrates cause weight gain and type 2 diabetes.

Most recreational endurance athletes who try low-carb diets do so for the same reasons that nonathletes do. Their main concern is not better performance but weight loss and better health. The problem is that carbohydrates per se do not, in fact, cause weight gain or type 2 diabetes. Athletes who go low-carb often do lose weight, but not for the reason they think, and in the process they lose fitness and performance capacity.

Advocates of low-carb diets for weight management and general health argue that carbohydrates cause weight gain by increasing insulin levels in the body. Insulin "traps" fat in fat cells, and, as a result, a high-carb diet causes more weight gain than a low-carb diet with the same number of total calories.

Except it doesn't. Science has never supported the insulin theory of weight gain, and the best and latest science emphatically contradicts it. For example, a 2015 study published in *Cell Metabolism* reported that a carefully controlled low-fat diet resulted in 68 percent more body fat loss than a low-carb diet of equal calories, even though the low-carb diet sharply reduced insulin levels.

So why do people tend to lose weight on low-carb diets? There are two main reasons. First, low-carb diets tend to be high-protein diets, and high-protein diets promote weight loss by increasing satiety and metabolism. But as I mentioned in Chapter 2, high-protein diets are not a good choice for endurance athletes and exercisers (at least not over the long term) because they impede the development of endurance fitness. The second reason people tend to lose weight on low-carb diets is that they usually eat fewer low-quality foods on such diets, and low-quality foods do cause weight gain.

Of the four low-quality food types, two—refined grains and sweets—are high in carbohydrates. These foods *are* fattening, and, unfortunately, they have given carbohydrates in general a bad reputation that extends unfairly to high-quality high-carb foods such as fruits and whole grains. The science is clear: fruits and whole grains promote a leaner body composition. Endurance athletes and exercisers who want to lose weight should continue to eat these foods, and perhaps even eat more of them, and reduce their consumption not only of the two high-carb low-quality food types but also of the other two low-quality food types: processed meat and seafood and fried foods. By doing so they will get leaner *and* fitter.

In 2015, researchers at the University of South Carolina reported that volunteers placed on a vegan diet for six months lost an average of 7.5 percent of their initial body weight without making any attempt to eat less. Carbohydrate intake actually *increased* on this diet. But, more importantly, diet quality increased alongside carb intake as the subjects replaced foods like pepperoni and ice cream with foods like brown rice and apples. The lesson of this study is not that a vegan diet is best for weight management but that the amount of carbohydrate in the diet is irrelevant to weight management. What matters is the quality of the food sources of carbohydrates and of the diet as a whole.

This principle is true with respect to type 2 diabetes as well. Although there is a proven link between the consumption of sugar-sweetened beverages and type 2 diabetes, there is no such link between carbohydrate consumption in general and the disease. Again, what matters is the quality of the foods that the carbs come from, not the quantity.

A carbohydrate-centered diet in itself is neither healthy nor unhealthy. What determines whether such a diet is healthy or unhealthy is whether the carbs come primarily from high-quality or low-quality sources. In the diets of elite Kenyan runners and other elite endurance athletes, carbs come predominantly from high-quality foods—particularly vegetables, fruits, whole grains, and milk. By contrast, in the United States and other industrialized countries, a sizable percentage of the total carbs in the diet comes from foods such as ice cream, potato chips, and pizza that also contain large amounts of fat, a combination that is rare in nature and proven to encourage overeating.

"Our carbohydrates are better because they are simple," Wilson Kipsang told me. "Yours come with a lot of extras."

During my time in Kenya, I discovered in a concrete and personal way how beneficial a high-quality, carb-centered diet can be for body composition. At home, my average daily Diet Quality Score is about 20 and I consume approximately 1,800 carbohydrate calories per day. In Kenya, my DQS jumped to 25 and my carbohydrate intake increased to 2,200 calories per day. These changes were almost unavoidable because low-quality foods just weren't available and all of the meals prepared for me were carb-centered.

The most memorable meal I ate in Kenya was served to me by a family of subsistence farmers living deep in the bush near the Kakamega rainforest. Every single item on my plate—ugali (high-carb), sukuma wiki, chapati (high-carb), mung beans, corn on the cob (high-carb), and chicken—was grown or raised on my hosts' property. Indeed, most of the plants and animals they came from had been living just hours before I ate them.

Not only did my diet change in Kenya, but my activity level did, too. At home, I normally spend about fourteen hours per week working out. In Kenya, I trained a lot less because the marathon I ran there fell in the middle of the trip, and it was necessary that I rest up beforehand and recover afterward. Despite my reduced activity level, and thanks to the high-quality carb-centered Kenyan diet, I lost 2.5 pounds and returned home lighter than I had been since high school.

Not All High-Carbohydrate Foods Are the Same

Table 5.1 shows just how different two diets supplying equal quantities of carbohydrates can be in terms of diet quality.

Practicing Habit 3

Emulating the elite athletes' habit of maintaining a carbohydrate-centered diet is a simple matter of including carbohydrate-rich foods in all meals and most snacks. This is not at all difficult to do for most people. Many foods that are normally eaten in each meal of the day are high in carbs. High-carb breakfast foods include oatmeal, bagels, and cold cereal. Some of the high-carb foods that are popular in the mid-day meal are bread, tortillas, and vegetable soups. At the dinner table,

Table 5.1   Two Diets with Same Quantity of Carbs Differ in Quality

Diet 1	Diet 2
Breakfast Glazed donut Starbucks Grande Caramel Macchiato	**Breakfast** Old-fashioned oatmeal with blueberries and almonds Orange juice Coffee with milk
Lunch Peanut butter and jelly Sandwich on white bread Milk chocolate bar Can of soda	**Lunch** Split pea soup Half of a turkey and veggie sandwich on whole wheat bread Tomato juice Apple
Dinner Spaghettios Canned peaches Sweetened iced tea	**Dinner** Brown rice with garlic and butter Two-bean pumpkin chili Red wine Peach
Carbohydrate Percentage	
67	69
Diet Quality Score	
-24	+28

potatoes and grains such as rice and quinoa fit the bill. Fruit and yogurt are among the high-carb foods that work well as snacks.

In practicing Habit 3, be sure to integrate it with the other four habits of the Endurance Diet. Combining Habit 3 with Habit 1, eating everything, means eating a wide variety of carbohydrate-rich foods. The typical American gets the vast majority of his or her carbohydrate calories from just three sources: corn, soy, and wheat. If you're thinking, "Wait: I don't eat much corn and soy," in fact, you probably do—you just eat them as highly processed ingredients of other foods. In any case, it's smart to branch out and get more of your carbs from other grains (amaranth, buckwheat, bulgur, millet, oats, quinoa, rice, sorghum, teff) and also from other carbohydrate-rich foods such as starchy vegetables and fruits.

We have already touched on the importance of combining the habit of maintaining a carbohydrate-centered diet with Habit 2 of the Endurance Diet: eating quality. Try to consistently get most of your carbs from high-quality foods and few of them from low-quality refined grains (e.g., white rice), sweets (e.g., pastries), and fried foods (e.g., French fries).

Combining Habit 3 with Habit 4—eating enough—is all you need to do to ensure you get the right *amount* of carbohydrates. As I mentioned above, the more you exercise, the more carbohydrates you must consume to maximize the benefits you get from your training. Eating enough is all about basing the amount of food you eat on your true energy needs as expressed through hunger and satiety. If you do this, you will naturally eat more as you train more and your energy needs increase. And if you're already on a carbohydrate-centered diet, your carb intake will automatically increase as your overall eating does, ensuring that you get enough.

Counting carbohydrate grams or calories is not particularly useful because there are no clear targets to aim for. Scientists have been unable to identify precise quantitative daily carbohydrate requirements for individual athletes based on training volume or overall energy expenditure. What they have found is that, in general, athletes with moderate training loads (up to two hours of exercise per day, depending on the type and intensity of training) who consume 5 to 7 grams of carbs per kilogram of body weight per day perform worse when they eat less carbohydrate but no better when they eat more, and that athletes with heavy training loads (over two hours per day, give or take) who consume 7 to 10 g/kg daily perform worse when they eat less but no better when they eat more.

Athletes who eat carb-centered diets and who consistently consume enough total calories in a day usually achieve these carb intake levels without tallying grams or calories, and indeed elite endurance athletes rarely do keep count. Nevertheless, it can be a worthwhile exercise to calculate your carbohydrate intake for one or two days immediately after you've shifted to carb-centered eating to see if it falls within the appropriate range. Food labels, online resources, and various smartphone apps can help with this. If your carb intake is low, and if you find yourself struggling to handle training loads you feel you ought to be able to handle, try adding more high-quality carbohydrate-rich foods to your diet.

Finally, it is important to practice Habit 3 of the Endurance Diet in combination with Habit 5: eating individually. To eat individually is to tailor your diet to meet your individual needs and preferences. One aspect of this process of customization is paying attention to how particular foods and eating patterns affect you and modifying those patterns accordingly. Although a carbohydrate-centered diet is generally best for endurance athletes and exercisers, not all high-carb foods agree with all of them. You may need to experiment a little to find a combination of foods that works optimally for you.

Even some of the world's best endurance athletes encounter personal restrictions of this sort. An extreme case is that of the American triathlete Amanda Stevens. Throughout her life, Stevens suffered from a "mystery illness" with a variety of symptoms, including intestinal bleeding, that were mostly gastrointestinal in nature. These symptoms became worse and worse until Stevens was forced to stop training and racing and seek help from specialists. She learned that she had celiac disease and was allergic to more than one hundred foods, a list that encompassed many of the carbohydrate sources that celiacs, who cannot eat wheat, often turn to, such as quinoa.

There are many recreational endurance athletes who, had they been in Stevens's place, would have gone on a low-carb diet. But Stevens knew she could not afford to do that, as it would have left her unable to perform at an elite level even if it did resolve her symptoms. So Stevens set about identifying the few carbohydrate-rich foods she could tolerate. There weren't many: red potatoes, yellow potatoes, russet potatoes, rice, and bananas. In order to meet the carbohydrate requirements imposed by the heavy training load demanded by Stevens's goal of winning major triathlons, she began to eat these foods with great frequency while avoiding all of her problem foods. In the next big race she did after making these changes, Stevens joined the exclusive sub-nine-hour Ironman club, winning the 2014 Ironman Arizona in 8:52:31.

If you ever find yourself thinking that a carbohydrate-centered diet can't work for you, imagine you're a professional endurance athlete and you *have* to make a carb-centered diet work for you in order to sustain your livelihood. If you do, you will almost certainly find that you can make it work, one way or another.

I see this happen often in the carbophobic athletes and exercisers I am able to persuade to take a chance on Habit 3. One example is Arwen, an ultrarunner from Utah. Like Amanda Stevens, Arwen suffered from digestive problems. After undergoing intestinal surgery in 2011, she found that a low-carb diet seemed to agree with her. Two years later, Arwen discovered she had a wheat allergy and responded by not only eliminating wheat from her diet but also by reducing her grain intake generally.

Although these challenges were particular to her, the carbophobic ethos of the culture she lived in contributed to a general conclusion that carbs are bad, so when Arwen got more serious about her training and racing, she remained on a low-carb diet. The surprising results were weight gain and premature fatigue in longer workouts. When Arwen came to me for help, I encouraged her to increase her carbohydrate intake, not by going back to eating foods that disagreed with her digestive system but rather by identifying carb-rich foods that she tolerated well. Over time, she compiled a list that included quinoa, beets, parsnips, brown rice, and sweet and white potatoes. Within weeks of increasing her carbohydrate intake, Arwen lost 5 pounds and experienced a significant energy increase in her workouts.

Happy endings like these are available to all carbophobic athletes who are willing to take a chance on carbs in an individual way in their pursuit of a solution to whatever is standing as an obstacle to the health and fitness results they seek.

6   Habit 4: Eat Enough

In SEPTEMBER 1972, FRANK SHORTER WON THE OLYMPIC MARATHON IN Munich, inspiring thousands of his fellow Americans to become runners. Three months later, Shorter won the Fukuoka Marathon in Japan, inspiring (among others, presumably) a thirteen-year-old boy named Nobuya "Nobby" Hashizume from the city of Tsu, near Nagoya, to become a runner. In the ensuing years, Hashizume developed into a pretty decent track athlete, posting a time of 15:12 for 5000 meters in college. His true destiny, however, was to coach other runners.

In Japan, professional running is dominated by corporate teams. Many of the country's major corporations employ rosters of elite runners. The athletes work a couple of hours a day in low-level office jobs, live together in a dormitory, are fed and coached by full-time company employees, and represent the company at team relay road races, called Ekiden, that are hugely popular in Japan, as well as in other events.

In 1989, Nobby Hashizume was offered his dream job. A major manufacturer of consumer electronics had just created a women's professional running team and Hashizume, now in his late twenties, was offered the position of assistant coach. Like most Japanese corporate teams, this one was very well funded. Hashizume and the head coach he worked under were paid executive salaries. The company built a dormitory with a fully equipped kitchen for the athletes and hired two chefs and a nutritionist to feed them. The new team brought on a pair of runners in its first year of existence and expanded to eight runners the following year.

Hashizume became disillusioned very quickly, however. The problem was his boss, who micromanaged the diet of the runners in a way that deeply troubled his young assistant. Ignoring the nutritionist's input, the head coach told the team chef exactly how many calories of food to prepare for each runner. It was never enough, yet the coach exacerbated the shortfall by standing sentinel in the refectory at mealtimes and telling the runners when to put down their chopsticks.

The best runner on the team was a naturally stocky young woman nicknamed Bebe. She loved to eat and, according Hashizume, the more she ate, the better she ran. But the head coach pressured her so relentlessly to reduce her food intake that Bebe eventually quit the team in protest. Hashizume himself quit after three years. He told me his greatest professional regret is that he didn't do more to protect the runners before he left.

In Hashizume's defense, the systematic undernourishment of distance runners was pervasive in Japan at the time. Indeed, runners everywhere have been susceptible to eating too little. Because the sport of running favors a low body weight and a lean body composition, runners who live and eat together often feel pressured to lose weight and to eat less as a means of losing weight. This pressure tends to be especially strong among female runners, who, quite apart from recognizing the performance advantages of being lean, are steeped in popular expectations to look skinny for the sake of being considered attractive. And the pressure is often intensified when female runners train under a male coach.

Within the Japanese corporate running teams of the 1980s, the pressure to undereat may have been magnified further by an especially pronounced emphasis on leanness, a relative dearth of reliable information about sports nutrition, and a tradition of respect for authority that made it difficult for athletes to speak up for their own interests when those interests clashed with a coach's will. This perfect storm of factors led to episodes that were even more unfortunate than the premature end of Bebe's professional running career.

Among the more infamous cases was that of Yumi Kokamo, who joined a corporate team in 1991, when she was just eighteen years old. One year later, Kokamo won the Osaka Ladies Marathon in 2:26:26, setting a new Japanese national record and a women's debut marathon world record. But her immense promise was never fulfilled. Her coach at the time was notorious for limiting athletes' food intake, and under his influence Kokamo "came very close to becoming anorexic," according to Hashizume. She struggled to a twenty-ninth-place finish in the 1992 Olympic Marathon, quit the team soon thereafter, and never regained her past form, retiring at age twenty-six.

The silver lining to tragedies like this one is that they taught runners and coaches that strictly limiting food intake sabotages endurance fitness. But this discovery alone was not enough to precipitate change. A positive counterexample was also needed. Fortunately, international travel exposed Japanese athletes and coaches to foreign athletes who did not artificially restrict the amount of food they ate but instead allowed internal signals of hunger and satiety to govern their intake. This practice, which defines the Endurance Diet habit of eating enough, is the only reliable way for people who engage in vigorous daily cardio exercise to avoid eating either too little (more common among highly competitive athletes) or too much (more common among less competitive athletes and noncompetitive exercisers). Encountering and interacting with athletes who ate enough and who performed better because they ate enough led Japanese athletes to do the same, and today nearly all elite Japanese endurance athletes, like elite athletes everywhere, practice this habit.

A good example of how this cross-pollination of best practices unfolded is the story of Misato Takagi, a triathlete who came to the United States from Japan in 2009 to train with an international group of elite triathletes coached by former world champion Siri Lindley in Boulder, Colorado. In her new environment, Takagi noticed two things. One was that the other athletes ate a lot more than she did. The other was that she couldn't keep up with those same athletes on long bike rides. It didn't take long for Takagi to put two and two together and realize that she couldn't keep up with her new training partners *because* she didn't eat as much.

A veteran of the Japanese corporate team system, Takagi was accustomed to worrying about and trying to avoid eating too much. In Boulder, without coaches looking over her shoulder at meals, she started to listen to her body and allow its appetite signals to determine how much food she ate. Takagi's newly acquired habit of eating enough carried her to a number of successes, including a victory at the 2010 Mazatlan ITU Pan American Cup and a runner-up finish in the following year's Roatlan ITU Pan American Cup. Takagi now coaches other triathletes back home in Japan, and she encourages all of them to trust their own appetite to ensure that their bodies are properly fueled for maximum performance.

Through many cross-cultural interactions like this one, Japan's elite endurance athletes have largely caught up to their competitors from other nations in practicing the fourth habit of the Endurance Diet. I saw this for myself in August 2015, when I spent five days as an observer at a training camp for five members of the Mitsui-Sumitomo women's running team (including 2:19:41 marathoner Yoko Shibui) in Boulder. The camp was hosted by none other than Nobby Hashizume, who after leaving his "dream job" in 1991 married an American woman and emigrated to the United States, and cohosted by Lorraine Moller, a New Zealand expatriate who won five marathons in Japan in the 1980s and 1990s and has maintained her Japan connection ever since.

On my first evening with the team, Hashizume and Moller, who are partners in a coaching certification business called the Lydiard Foundation, held a potluck dinner at Moller's home. It was attended by all five Japanese runners, their head coach Shigeharu Watanabe, and their assistant coach Takashi Hayashi, and several luminaries from the Boulder running community, including Mike Sandrock, who covers the sport for the *Boulder Daily Camera*, and John Elliott, founder of marathonguide.com and owner of a house located three doors down from Moller's, where the Mitsui-Sumitomo runners stayed.

The Japanese contingent contributed a curry dish and rice to the occasion. Other guests brought chicken breasts, corn on the cob, quinoa salad, a mixed-greens salad, and watermelon. The Mitsui-Sumitomo runners sampled all of it. Although this might not seem like a big deal, Hashizume assured me the occasion represented a major change from the bad old days, when Japanese running teams that came to America for altitude training would go out of their way to avoid interacting with the natives and eating their food.

The next morning, Hashizume cooked French toast for the runners. He did so at the special request of Shibui, who had eaten Hashizume's French toast previously at a training camp in Flagstaff in 2009. Shibui has beefy legs for an elite runner and gains weight easily. One of her goals for the three-week training stint in Boulder was to lose a bit of fat and get down to her competition weight of 104 pounds (Shibui is five feet three). Yet her breakfast on that morning consisted of four slices of French toast plus a salad and an iced coffee. I did the math and concluded that the whole meal came to roughly 1,000 calories.

Why did Yoko Shibui eat 1,000 calories at breakfast when she was trying to lose weight? Because she wasn't trying to lose weight for the sake of dropping a dress size; she was trying to lose weight to run faster, and she understood that she would only run faster if she lost weight the right way—not by restricting her food intake but by training for peak fitness and giving her body the fuel it needed to get the most benefit out of her training. Coach Watanabe watched approvingly as Shibui took a second helping of Hashizume's famous French toast.

"I personally don't think it's a very good idea to lose too much weight," Watanabe told me, with Hashizume acting as translator.

Later, I quizzed the runners directly about their attitudes and practices relating to the quantity of food they ate.

"How do you know if you're eating the right amount of food from day to day?" I asked Yuki Hidaka, a 10,000-meter specialist with a personal-best time of 32:10.

"I eat until I'm satisfied," she answered through Hashizume.

I pressed this point with Yuri Nozoe, the youngest member of the team at age nineteen, who was also trying to lose weight.

"Do you really trust your appetite to tell you when you've had enough to eat but not too much?" I asked.

"I trust it more than I trust my eyes!" she answered with a laugh, meaning (Hashizume explained) that she trusted her body's appetite signals more than she did any preconceived *idea* about how much she should eat.

Most of the meals that the Mitsui-Sumitomo runners ate in Boulder consisted of simple, traditional Japanese foods prepared in a secondary kitchen in Moller's house by coach Watanabe or by a local Japanese physical therapist hired for the camp. Breakfast was usually miso soup, rice, eggs, and salad. For lunch and dinner the runners ate rice and sautéed vegetables with chicken, pork, or ground beef, or else more Japanese curry (a team favorite). But on the team's last night in Boulder, their hosts took them out to eat at an Italian restaurant on Pearl Street along with several American guests.

No sooner had our party of sixteen been seated than Coach Watanabe and assistant coach Hayashi ordered beers. This was a signal to their runners that they should feel free to eat whatever they wanted, and they did. Hidaka and Kana Orino (a marathon specialist with a personal best of 2:33:51) each ordered a plate of pasta and also split a small pizza and a salad. Having dispatched these items, they finished off another pizza that had been ordered by the two children in our group.

At this point in the feast, a two-foot extendable fork was produced from somewhere. The runners and some of the others began using it to steal bits of food from plates on the opposite side of the table. Before long they were using the same implement to feed others at long range. Such silliness did much to overcome the barrier of language (only Hashizume was fluent in both English and Japanese). Indeed, the group became so rowdy and made such a mess that I feared we would be kicked out of the restaurant. In the end, though, we left of our own volition and walked two doors down to a gelato shop for dessert.

Hashizume told me afterward that he sent photos of the gathering to two of his former corporate team runners who had been on the brink of developing eating disorders under the head coach's strict rule. Both expressed shock at how much things had changed and envy for the healthy, carefree relationship with food that now existed in at least some Japanese running teams.

These teams were among the last dominoes to fall in the global spread of the habit of eating enough among elite endurance athletes. Today, virtually all of the world's top racers trust their internal appetite signals to govern how much they eat. This was demonstrated by the answers I received from elite athletes to a handful of questions included in my research questionnaire that were intended to ascertain whether elite athlete respondents practiced the habit of eating enough. For example, in response to the question, "Are you more concerned about making sure you eat enough or about avoiding eating too much?" Icelandic cross-country skier Sævar Birgisson wrote, "When I am training a lot I just eat as much as I can, to have enough energy to get through the training. But when I'm training less I eat less."

Responses like this one indicate that elite endurance athletes neither restrain their eating nor overeat but simply allow their activity level to affect their appetite and their appetite to govern how much food they eat.

Eating Enough versus Restrained Eating

You may be wondering how this applies to nonelite athletes and exercisers. The amount of food that any endurance athlete or exerciser eats from day to day has as much effect on fitness and performance as the types of food he or she eats. The goal is balance: to eat enough food to fuel maximum performance in training but not so much that excess body fat accumulates or is retained. Elite endurance athletes maintain this balance by paying mindful attention to their appetite—that is, by practicing the habit of eating enough.

Recreational endurance athletes and exercisers often eat less than enough or more than enough rather than precisely enough as the elites do. Overeating is more common than undereating among nonelite endurance athletes and exercisers, just as it is generally in affluent populations. But undereating is by no means rare among people who engage in daily cardio exercise. It happens in part because endurance training increases energy needs and in part because some athletes and exercisers, like the elite female Japanese runners of the recent past, mistakenly view eating less as the best way to get leaner. Seriously competitive athletes are the most prone to undereat, and the consequences of undereating are severest for those who train hardest.

The reason recreational endurance athletes and exercisers so often eat too little or too much is that they don't emulate the elites' habit of regulating their food intake through mindful attention to appetite signals representing their true energy needs. Undereating typically results from *dietary restraint*, or intentionally defying the body's hunger signals. But undereating itself often leads to reactive overeating. The more common cause of overeating, however, is *mindless eating*, or allowing food temptations to override satiety signals telling a person that he or she has already had enough to eat. In this section and in the next one I will explain the nature and consequences of dietary restraint and mindless eating, respectively. Later in the chapter I will explain how to avoid and overcome both eating restraint and mindless eating by learning (or, more accurately, *re*learning) how to practice the Endurance Diet habit of eating mindfully to eat enough.

Esther Waugh of Stanford University has defined restrained eating as "the conscious attempt to limit and monitor food intake to achieve or maintain a desired weight." There are two basic styles of restrained eating. Some restrained eaters make a conscious choice to eat a certain amount of food each day (often measured in calories) and limit themselves to that amount of food regardless of how hungry they are. Others practice a feel-based version of restrained eating in which they pay attention to their hunger but intentionally eat less than necessary to satisfy it.

Some experts believe that restrained eating is a natural adaptive response to an environment in which overeating is all too easy and common. But not everyone who lives in a fattening environment has this response, and in fact the healthiest and fittest people in such environments, including elite endurance athletes, tend not to be highly restrained eaters. These observations have led other experts, including Jaime Silva of Frontera University in Chile, to conclude that restrained eating is the product of a "dysfunctional emotional regulatory system" in certain individuals. This does not mean that people who try to regulate their food intake through dietary restraint are head cases. It just means they tend to share a particular coping style that leads them to "solve" the problem of overeating or being too heavy by adopting a general intent to eat less than they want to.

The personality trait that is most closely associated with restrained eating is low self-esteem. It doesn't take a PhD in psychology to understand why. As a weight-control method, restrained eating entails repeated self-denial, a systematic tuning-out and thwarting of the body's wants that is based on an implicit belief that the body's wants cannot be trusted. Day after day, meal after meal, the restrained eater says "no" to the types and/or amounts of food he or she would like to eat. It is not inaccurate to describe this pattern as essentially masochistic.

Regardless of where it comes from, restrained eating doesn't work very well. Although you might assume that restrained eating causes people to undereat, it is actually more often linked with overeating. One reason is that dietary restraint is in many cases a response to a preexisting tendency to overeat. In other words, people who are prone to overeat develop a generalized intent to resist this predisposition. But this response fails to result in less overeating in the long term because eating less than one wants is psychologically taxing. In essence, it drains willpower, leaving the restrained eater more vulnerable to the very temptations he or she is trying to resist. Studies have demonstrated that individuals who exhibit high levels of eating restraint have a lower ability to resist certain food treats. They are also more prone to food binges. A person who intentionally undereats today is therefore more likely to overeat tomorrow.

When dietary restraint does work, it tends to work all too well. Research has shown that men and women who exhibit the very highest levels of eating restraint are likely to become anorexic or bulimic. Endurance athletes and exercisers who develop eating disorders face consequences that go beyond those experienced by less active people, among them frequent injury. But even in the absence of an eating disorder, eating even slightly too little generates negative outcomes for endurance fitness seekers.

Studies indicate that a typical inactive person can reduce his or her normal daily calorie intake by as much as 30 percent and suffer no negative health effects—and perhaps even experience health improvements—as long as diet quality remains consistently high. In a 2013 review of past research on medically supervised calorie restriction, for example, scientists at Washington University School of Medicine concluded that "moderate calorie restriction with adequate nutrition has a powerful protective effect against obesity, type 2 diabetes, inflammation, hypertension, [and] cardiovascular disease and reduces metabolic risk factors associated with cancer" and "improves markers of cardiovascular aging."

The story is very different for endurance athletes and exercisers, however. Vigorous daily cardio exercise itself offers powerful protection against obesity, type 2 diabetes, inflammation, hypertension, cardiovascular disease, cancer, and aging. Calorie restriction offers no additional protection to people with a high level of endurance fitness. Instead it creates other problems by failing to supply the body with the raw materials it needs to absorb and adapt to the stress of training. The most common consequences of undereating in endurance athletes and exercisers are lethargy, poor workout performance, slow postworkout recovery, increased cold and flu risk, and loss of muscle mass. Restrained eaters also suffer more overuse injuries. A 2008 study by researchers at San Diego State University reported a strong correlation between restrained eating and low bone mineral density—a risk factor for stress fractures—in adolescent female runners.

The most surprising outcome of restrained eating in endurance athletes and exercisers is weight gain. I see this happen most often in athletes who restrain their eating through calorie targets. An example is Wendy, a runner from Spokane, Washington, who began counting calories (or "points") in 2011 as a member of Weight Watchers. Three years later, she was 18 pounds lighter and happy with the program. But then Wendy decided to train for her first marathon. Believing that additional weight loss would enable her to run better, she continued to eat 1,300 calories per day and was stunned when the needle on her bathroom scale began to move in the wrong direction.

Wendy's surprise is understandable. Weight gain resulting from eating too little seems to defy the laws of mathematics. Yet it is quite common in people who exercise a lot. The reason is that the combination of low energy supply and high activity levels creates a type of stress that causes the body to protectively slow its metabolism. In a 2014 study published in the *Scandinavian Journal of Medicine & Science in Sports*, researchers at the University of Copenhagen found that high-level female endurance athletes with low energy availability (the scientific term for inadequate calorie intake, which in this case was defined as fewer than 45 calories per kilogram of fat-free body mass per day) had a resting metabolic rate that was 6.8 percent lower than that of their peers with adequate energy intake. The same metabolic slowing phenomenon is partly responsible for weight regain in dieters who initially lose weight, including, as one study found, former contestants on the reality television program *The Biggest Loser*.

Setting a higher calorie target is not the best solution to the problem of weight gain resulting from calorie targets that are too low. There is no formula that athletes and exercisers can use to precisely determine how many calories they need to fuel their training optimally without impeding progress toward (or maintenance of) their optimal body composition. The underlying physiology is too complex. Plus, it's a moving target, because energy needs change daily with fluctuations in training. The true solution to weight gain and other consequences of low calorie targets is to abandon calorie targets altogether and replace them with the feel-based approach to regulating food intake that elite athletes use. Only the body's own appetite control system is sensitive enough to guide athletes and exercisers to precisely the right amount of eating.

When I work with athletes whose restrained eating has caused them to gain weight and/or lose energy, I teach them to replace calorie targets with appetite-based eating, and it works. One such athlete is Amanda, a runner and triathlete from San Diego. Before she started to train for her first half marathon, Amanda restricted herself to 2,000 calories per day. After she started to train for her first marathon, she continued to eat 2,000 calories per day. Six weeks into her training, Amanda stepped on a scale and was horrified to see that she had put on 6 pounds in that short span of time.

I advised Amanda to stop counting calories and start trusting her appetite. She did so and three weeks later she was back down to her original weight. What's more, the fatigue that had begun to accumulate over the first six weeks of her training and that she had thought was normal dissipated, and her workouts improved.

The scientific term for the skill that elite endurance athletes and others rely on to eat the right amount of food by feel is *appetite awareness*. Everyone possesses this skill, but in restrained eaters it has become somewhat rusty from disuse. Fortunately, clinical research backs my observation that even the most restrained eaters can learn to reconnect with their body's signals and enjoy the benefits of eating enough. In a 2010 study, for example, psychologists at Emory University tested the effects of appetite awareness training on individuals with disordered eating. They found that those who showed the most improvement in appetite awareness also exhibited the greatest improvement in disordered eating symptoms.

Interestingly, the same solution works for people who habitually ignore their body's appetite signals in the opposite direction, overeating by eating mindlessly.

Eating Enough versus Mindless Eating

For every endurance athlete or exerciser like Amanda or Wendy whose weight gain is caused by eating too little, there are many more whose weight gain is caused by eating too much. A majority of people in affluent societies today, including most endurance fitness seekers, overeat. Seventy percent of American adults currently meet the medical standard for being considered overweight, and nobody becomes over-weight without overeating. Ours is a society of overeaters.

Endurance athletes and exercisers are somewhat less likely than sedentary persons to overeat because they burn more calories through activity and therefore must eat more in order to eat too much. But overeating is still very common among recreational endurance fitness seekers. According to a 2009 scientific survey that I helped administer, 54 percent of competitive endurance athletes are dissatisfied with their current weight.

The typical endurance athlete or exerciser who weighs more than he or she would like to does not count calories or measure portion sizes but instead eats by feel. This has given rise to a widespread belief that appetite cannot be trusted to properly regulate food intake—that a person who allows feelings of hunger and satiety to govern how much food he or she eats is certain to eat too much. The flaw in this assumption is that it conflates two distinct types of hunger: physical and hedonic.

Physical hunger is the set of cues the body uses to communicate a real and present need for food. The major cues are a hollow feeling in the stomach and a strong desire to eat. Hedonic hunger is a desire to eat that occurs in the absence of physical hunger and is often brought about by the presence of tempting foods. Brian Wansink of Cornell University has coined the term *mindless eating* to refer to eating hedon-ically, without paying attention to, or without properly interpreting, the body's hunger and satiety signals. The Endurance Diet habit of eating enough entails eating only when one is physically hungry and only enough to satisfy physical hunger. In other words, it entails eat-ing mindfully versus mindlessly. Most people who regulate their food intake by feel eat to satisfy hedonic hunger on top of physical hunger. This habit of mindless eating is why they overeat and why they mis-takenly believe they cannot rely on their appetite to properly regulate the amount of food they eat.

In fact, the body's built-in appetite regulatory system works perfectly well in most people. The problem is the modern food environment in which this system is forced to operate. In this environment, people are continuously bombarded with temptations to eat more than they need to—and particularly to eat highly palatable and fattening low-quality foods. These temptations are hard to resist and most people do not resist them successfully, even when they think they do. For example, if you see a television advertisement for a fast-food restaurant at which you never eat, you may assume that the commercial has not influenced you. But studies have shown that people who see such ads are more likely to eat low-quality foods they already have at home, regardless of whether they ever eat the specific foods advertised.

Evidence that environment rather than appetite is to blame for our overeating comes from studies of nonindustrialized cultures where fast food and fast-food advertising are lacking. In 1982, Jonathan Fried-laender and John Rhoads of Harvard University looked at patterns of change in weight and body composition among adults in six different populations in the Solomon Islands and Papua New Guinea with different degrees of exposure to modern industrialized societies. The researchers found that men and women with the least such exposure tended to gain no weight and very little body fat throughout adulthood, whereas those with the most exposure gained significant amounts of weight and body fat. Obviously, all of these people possessed the same built-in appetite control system. What differed was their environment.

Additional proof that the body's built-in appetite control system is able to properly regulate food intake is found in research on the effects of exercise on appetite. Physical activity is the primary variable affecting energy needs. If appetite is an accurate indicator of energy needs, it should be highly sensitive to changes in activity level, and indeed it is. Dozens of studies have demonstrated that working out has both immediate and long-term effects on hormones involved in appetite control and on appetite itself and eating behavior.

A final bit of proof that appetite *can* be trusted to properly control the amount of food we eat comes from studies of children. Very young children do not overeat. Research has shown that when infants are fed less often, they consume larger portions, and when they are fed more often, they consume smaller portions. But toddlers tend to consume the same portion sizes regardless of how often they eat. By this stage they have already been trained to regulate their food intake by external cues instead of internal ones.

Fortunately, other research has demonstrated that the capacity to eat mindfully can be restored at any age. Infants ask to be fed when they experience cues of physical hunger, particularly a hollow feeling in the stomach. They stop feeding when they feel a comfortable fullness in the belly. Older children and adults often begin to eat in the absence of physical hunger cues and continue eating until they feel stuffed or the food is gone or both. But adults who reconnect with their body's signals are able to restore their ability to eat the right amount of food and lose excess body fat accumulated through habitual overeating.

In 2010, Mario Ciampolini and colleagues at Firenze University trained a mixed group of fifty-one overweight subjects and seventy-nine normal-weight subjects to recognize physical hunger and to distinguish it from hedonic hunger. An additional twenty-three overweight subjects and twenty-eight normal-weight subjects were used as controls and received no training (although they were given the same diet and physical activity recommendations as the trained subjects). After the training, the researchers found that the trained subjects' ratings of physical hunger were closely correlated with blood insulin levels, an objective marker of physical hunger.

In the next part of the experiment, the trained subjects were instructed to go home and eat only when they felt physical hunger. If a normal mealtime came around and they were not hungry, they had to wait until they were. The subjects were instructed also to adjust the composition and size of their meals so that physical hunger occurred predictably at normal mealtimes, thus minimizing the disruptiveness of appetite-based eating to their daily routine. After an initial adjustment period, the trained subjects consistently experienced physical hunger just before normal mealtimes.

At the end of the five-month study period, the trained overweight subjects had lost an average of 14.75 pounds. The reason was simply that they were no longer mindlessly eating when they did not need to or eating more than they needed to in order to satisfy their physical hunger. Trained normal-weight subjects lost an average of 5.5 pounds, indicating that they, too, had previously engaged in a certain amount of mindless eating. Normal-weight controls actually gained weight during the five-month study period, while overweight controls lost a small amount of weight (perhaps an effect of the diet and physical activity recommendations they had received).

Becoming conscious of the distinction between physical and hedonic hunger and developing a habit of eating to satisfy physical hunger works just as well to help endurance athletes and exercisers overcome overeating as it does with nonathletes. I see it happen all the time. A typical case is that of Maryse and her husband Marc, triathletes who began to practice the habit of eating enough after they heard me speak about the Endurance Diet at a triathlon conference in Canada. A few months later, Maryse contacted me to report that she had lost 10 pounds, and Marc, 30 pounds, and that both of them were fitter and racing better than ever.

How to Eat Enough

Practicing Habit 4 of the Endurance Diet requires only self-awareness and consistency. It does *not* require willpower, because eating enough means just that—eating enough to keep your physical hunger satisfied. It is only hedonic hunger that you must say "no" to.

If you've fallen out of the habit of paying mindful attention to your appetite—either through restrained eating or through mindless eating—you can relearn it fairly quickly by re-creating the experiment I described in the previous section. I recommend that you start on a weekend, when you have more freedom to eat at irregular times. If you wake up hungry on Saturday morning, go ahead and eat. If you don't, wait until you experience physical hunger. When you do eat, stop when you feel comfortably satisfied but not stuffed. After you've eaten your first meal of the day, wait until you are physically hungry again before you have your next meal.

On the second day, do the same thing, but adjust the size of your meals in an attempt to ensure that you are physically hungry at normal mealtimes. For example, if you were not physically hungry at your normal dinnertime on the first day, eat a lighter lunch on the second day. Adjusting the timing of your meals and adding or removing snacks from your normal routine are options as well. Use common sense in making these adjustments. For example, adding a midafternoon snack to your schedule makes more sense as a solution to getting hungry before dinnertime than does eating until you are stuffed at lunch.

You may also manipulate the composition of your meals, as the subjects in Ciampolini's experiment did, to influence the time course of your appetite. As a general rule, foods with high protein, water, and/ or fiber content are more satiating, but it's not always easy to predict a food's effect on satiety. I recommend that you consult the "Fullness Factor" ratings for individual foods on nutritiondata.com when planning these types of substitutions. Don't allow these ratings to become the primary determinant of what you eat, however. The composition of your meals should be determined mainly by Endurance Diet Habits 2 (eating quality) and 3 (eating carb-centered). You should never lower your diet quality or risk failing to consume enough carbohydrate for the sake of micromanaging your appetite.

When you return to your normal weekday routine, continue the process of adjusting the size, and perhaps also the timing, frequency, and composition of your meals and snacks so that physical hunger symptoms return shortly before normal mealtimes with greater and greater predictability. Don't drive yourself crazy trying to achieve perfection in this effort. The main purpose of the exercise is to make you a more mindful eater generally. Once you are attuned to the signals of your body's real energy needs, it is quite easy to eat the right amount of food day in and day out.

If you're currently a restrained eater, you may need to repeat the mindful eating experiment a few times before eating enough becomes habitual. In a 2007 study involving college women at risk for eating disorders, Arnica Buckner of the University of Colorado found that appetite awareness training yielded immediate improvements in restrained eating, but that these improvements were greatly diminished after one month. As I stated above, practicing Habit 4 successfully requires not just awareness but also *consistency.*

If you're currently prone to mindless eating, beware of temptation situations in which overeating is most likely to occur. Following are five specific situations where being mindful of the distinction between physical and hedonic hunger will be most helpful to you.

Portion Distortion

The phrase "portion distortion" refers to the mismatch between the meal sizes that are sufficient to satisfy our true energy needs and those we habitually choose. Self-selected portions are strongly influenced by our environment. What we consider a normal portion size is affected by the portion sizes we were served at home as children, by how much the people around us eat, and by restaurant and packaged food portion sizes. Research has demonstrated that portion sizes of restaurant menu items, packaged foods, and home-prepared meals began to increase in the early 1970s in the United States and continued to grow through the late 1990s.

Were Americans not eating enough to satisfy their physical hunger before the 1970s? Obviously, they were. The difference is that we are eating far beyond our physical needs today. A key part of overcoming mindless overeating is learning to choose portions that are just big enough to keep physical hunger at bay until shortly before the next mealtime.

Plate Cleaning

It is almost impossible to completely avoid excessive portion sizes. If you eat out with any regularity, it's only a matter of time before a server gives you a plate containing more food than you need. This wouldn't be a problem if people did not have a learned tendency to "clean their plate," but they do. A survey by the American Institute of Cancer Research reported that 69 percent of Americans finish their restaurant entrees most of the time or always. Of this 69 percent, three-fifths rated restaurant portions as "just right in size," but these subjective ratings can't be trusted because other research has shown that when people are served smaller portions they eat less without feeling any less satisfied.

If you habitually clean your plate, it's important that you eat especially mindfully whenever you eat out or are served a meal that may be bigger than you need. Eat at a measured pace, listen to your body, and put the fork down when you are comfortably full, no matter how much food is left. If you don't want to waste food, box it up and save it for later.

Spontaneous Eating

As the name suggests, spontaneous eating is eating without prior planning, when a temptation or opportunity arises. An example is walking into a business meeting in a conference room where a selection of fresh pastries is available and partaking of them even though you ate breakfast 90 minutes earlier.

You can reduce the likelihood of giving in to temptation in such situations by keeping them from catching you off guard. Of course, you can't predict exactly when a Girl Scout will ring your doorbell and offer cookies, but you can adopt a general expectation that spontaneous eating opportunities will arise and recognize them for what they are. It also helps to know ahead of time what you will do when they arise. Psychologists call this type of plan an implementation intention.

The strictest plan you might have for spontaneous eating is to say "no" in all cases except when you are physically hungry and when eating the specific food you're tempted with won't spoil your Diet Quality Score for the day. But who wants to say "no" to a Girl Scout? A less strict option is to turn spontaneous eating opportunities into planned eating occasions by saving the food temptation for later. Another compromise is to allow yourself to sample food temptations—for example, cut a bite-size piece off one of those delicious honey buns on the conference table.

Distracted Eating

It's a fact: people eat more when their attention is on something other than food, whether it's a television show, a website, or even a dinner table conversation. I would never recommend eating alone when you could eat with others as a way to avoid mindless overeating, but I do recommend eliminating technological distractions. If you just have to eat your dinner in front of the TV, mitigate the distraction effect by preparing an appropriate portion size and putting any leftovers away before you sit down to eat.

Emotional Eating

Some of us eat more, or make less healthy food choices, when we're anxious, stressed, or unhappy. Mindfulness can help here to some degree. When strong emotions cause you to crave ice cream, pause to listen to your body. If it's not giving you physical hunger signals, try to find a healthier outlet for your emotion, whether it's exercise, social contact, creative expression, or something else. If you are hungry, try to find something healthier to eat. It helps when low-quality food temptations aren't in your home in the first place.

Such advice is easier to accept than to apply for people with strong emotional eating tendencies, who know perfectly well they're not hungry when anxiety, stress, or sadness causes them to reach for the ice cream container. Counseling is often the best answer in these cases. Working with a trained mental health professional to address the underlying issues that predispose you toward emotional eating may not only give you better skills for dealing with negative emotions but may also make you a less anxious, less stressed, and happier person.

Advice for Those Seeking to Lose Weight

Habit 4 of the Endurance Diet applies to everyone whose current primary goal is maximizing endurance fitness. It does not apply to people whose current primary goal is losing excess body fat. That's because these two goals are incompatible. Although people who follow the Endurance Diet in pursuit of maximum endurance fitness do tend to get leaner, the *fastest* way to lose excess body fat is to maintain a substantial daily energy deficit by restricting food intake, a measure that tends to compromise the benefits of intensive training.

If losing weight is currently more important to you than attaining peak fitness, you should complete a weight-loss focus phase, something that even some elite endurance athletes do to reverse off-season weight gain, before fully adopting the Endurance Diet. Two of the five habits of the Endurance Diet—eating carb-centered meals and allowing appetite to govern the amount of food you eat—are excluded from the diet I recommend for weight-loss focus phases. In Chapter 9, I will fully explain how to execute a weight-loss focus phase.

7   Habit 5: Eat Individually

A WELCOME MAT POSITIONED OUTSIDE THE FRONT ENTRANCE OF THE PAINT-box Lodge in Canmore, Alberta, Canada, identifies the establishment as "Olympian-Owned." The Olympians it refers to are Sara Renner and Thomas Grandi, who opened the lodge in 2010 after retiring from their respective sports. Renner, a cross-country skier, won a world championships bronze medal for Canada in the individual sprint in 2005 and an Olympic silver medal in the team sprint in 2006. Grandi, who is Renner's husband, represented his native Italy in the giant slalom and slalom ski events at the Salt Lake City Games in 2002 and the Turin Games in 2006.

I checked into the Paintbox Lodge on a mild May afternoon in 2015. Renner has described the lodge's interior design aesthetic as "rustic meets modern," and I found this description to be accurate enough, except that the rustic and modern elements do not actually meet. The lobby and guest rooms are entirely rustic: wool carpets underfoot, exposed beams above, and pinewood walls decorated with local artwork all around. Only the kitchen is modern: clean white cabinetry, bright red splash tiles, and stainless steel Miele appliances. Although the Paintbox Lodge has just five guestrooms, the kitchen is outfitted for industrial use because it serves not only to feed guests but also as a venue for cooking classes.

Sara Renner and Thomas Grandi—Renner especially—are really into food and healthy eating. Over coffee, Renner explained to me that when she was a child her parents owned a backcountry guest lodge in western Alberta where all of the meals were made fresh from local ingredients. Renner herself was cooking by age seven. After leaving home as a teenager to ski professionally, she had no difficulty in feeding herself according to the same high standards of quality and taste she had become accustomed to. Renner believes that the same diet that fueled her to success in international racing is good for everyone. In fact, one of the cooking classes taught at Paintbox is called "Eat Like an Olympian." The instructor is Marcel Holzherr, who also serves as the chef for the Canadian national cross-country and alpine ski teams.

The class has been a hit among Canmore locals and visitors, and it has been a transformative experience for some. One of Holzherr's early students was Andrew Nickerson, head of Canmore's tourism board. In the four months after he took the class, Nickerson lost 35 pounds. He did so without conscious intent and without thinking of himself as "going on a diet." He just started cooking like Holzherr. A non-exerciser at the time he took the class, Nickerson felt so much more energetic after he changed his diet that he started walking to work every day.

In a phone conversation, I asked Holzherr what it means to eat like an Olympian. I knew the answer already, but I was gratified nevertheless when he described what I call the Endurance Diet. Holzherr believes in a well-rounded diet that includes all of the natural food types. Among his favorites in each category are kale, apples, olive oil, spelt, Coho salmon, and plain yogurt. He is also a big believer in food quality in the secondary sense of "high grade," recommending, for example, that in-season, organic, and locally sourced vegetables be chosen in preference to the alternatives whenever possible. Holzherr has no fear of carbohydrates, advising both athletes and everyday active people to enjoy carb-packed foods such as buckwheat pancakes with berries and bananas, mashed potatoes with carrot and cumin, and spelt pasta. And, on the topic of calories, Holzherr has little to say, believing that when people eat quality, the quantity of the food they eat tends to take care of itself.

That covers four of the five habits of the Endurance Diet. But what about the fifth: eating individually? Holzherr is a strong advocate of customizing the diet to fit personal needs and preferences. At events such as the 2014 Winter Olympics in Vancouver and the 2016 cross-country skiing World Cup in Canmore, he prepares meals for the entire Canadian cross-country and alpine ski teams. (At the latter event, he used the Paintbox Lodge's kitchen.) Understanding that each athlete has unique needs and preferences, he serves buffet-style, with enough options for everybody.

"When I look around the room, no two plates are exactly the same," he told me proudly.

Holzherr not only accommodates the individual needs and preferences of the men and women he works with but encourages athletes to actively discover what works best for them. He invites athletes to monitor their performance, their sleep, and even their stool in order to identify problems that could have a dietary solution. To get younger athletes started on this process, he sometimes takes them out to a local family restaurant for a relatively low-quality meal after they have adjusted to eating like Olympians. According the Holzherr, the athletes always feel terrible afterward, and that's the point. He wants them to be attuned to the differences that eating the right things and the wrong things makes in terms of how they feel and function.

"All of us need to be conscious eaters," he says.

Eating Like an Olympian

The morning after my arrival in Canmore, I made a short drive to the home of Devon Kershaw, a three-time Olympian and a fourteen-year member of the Canadian National Cross-Country Ski Team. When I arrived at 7:30 a.m. sharp, the thirty-two-year-old Ontario native was just preparing his first meal of the day.

It was not exactly a typical North American breakfast. Kershaw filled a plate with raw spinach, sliced red and yellow peppers, a few raspberries, strips of mango, and several slices of Bündnerfleisch, a Swiss cured meat. He wrapped the veggies in the meat and ate them like spring rolls. He also ate two slices of rye bread spread with butter and sugar-free strawberry jam and topped with a delicious Norwegian brown cheese. (I know it was delicious because he shared some with me.) He drank two cups of espresso and a glass of water.

Hunger satisfied, Kershaw changed into workout clothes and ran a half-mile straight uphill to the Canmore Nordic Centre. A uniquely Canadian phenomenon, the Nordic Centre is a collection of outdoor and indoor facilities—including cross-country ski trails, a biathlon shooting range, and a weight room—where elite winter sports athletes and members of the community at large train side by side. On this morning, Kershaw made his way directly to the weight room, where he performed two hours of mobility movements, core exercises, balance drills, and Olympic lifts with several teammates as coach Justin Wadsworth looked on.

I met up with Kershaw again at his home for lunch. Since I had last seen him, he had run back down the hill, eaten four spoonfuls of cottage cheese as a recovery snack, and immersed himself in a shelf-building project. His midday repast was a salad of mixed greens, kale, beetroot, red and yellow peppers, apple slices, avocado, olive oil, balsamic vinegar, Thai spice tuna, and cottage cheese. This eclectic mixture was supplemented with a couple more pieces of rye bread with butter and Gruyère cheese. He drank sparkling water.

At 3:15, Kershaw was eating again. His preafternoon workout snack consisted of more rye bread (with cheese and jam), a bit of plain yogurt with mango and raspberries, Bündnerfleisch, and a cortado (espresso with milk). By 4:30, he was back at the Nordic Centre. There he strapped on a pair of roller skis and spent an hour and a half cruising around a paved course designed especially for such use. His teammates, meanwhile, did a higher-intensity workout centered on a set of four, 10-minute efforts at lactate threshold intensity. Kershaw's 2014–2015 racing season had been wiped out by illness—a double-whammy of pneumonia and whooping cough—and he still wasn't quite ready for hard training. As soon as he finished skiing, he guzzled a bottle of carbohydrate–protein recovery drink.

After returning home, Kershaw set about preparing dinner. He had a friend coming over to dine with him, so he aimed to impress, serving thick-cut pork chops with caramelized onions and apples; roasted white potatoes and sweet potatoes with olive oil, garlic, and rosemary; homemade sourdough bread with pumpkin and flaxseeds topped with Gruyère cheese; and red wine.

After his friend left and before he went to bed, Kershaw ate one last time. He enjoyed one of his favorite evening snacks: muesli with yogurt, almonds, and fruit (specifically raspberries and mangoes, because that's what he had in the fridge).

The day I spent with Devon Kershaw was a very typical one for him, diet-wise. But he hadn't always eaten what I saw him eat. If I had spent a day with Kershaw when he was a young athlete still living in his parents' home, I would have observed some differences. For example, in those days he ate dessert (often homemade pie with ice cream) almost every night, but he does so much less frequently now.

If I had spent a day with Kershaw near the beginning of his professional career, I would have found that his diet looked more like his current one, but not exactly like it. For example, he used to take a lot of supplements during that period, whereas today his supplement use is minimal.

Kershaw's diet continues to evolve. If I had spent a day with the skier even two months earlier than I did, I would have seen some differences in his diet. At that time, he was still eating eggs for breakfast every morning, but he cut them out of his diet six weeks before I came to Canmore. (I'll share the reasons for this change and for the change in Kershaw's supplementation practices in the next section.)

The meals and snacks that Devon Kershaw ate under my watchful eye on a Tuesday in May were the outcomes of a long personal dietary evolution that will probably continue throughout his life. Like most elite endurance athletes, Kershaw eats consciously, to use Marcel Holzherr's term. Conscious eating encompasses but extends beyond mindful eating, as discussed in Chapter 6. Eating mindfully entails listening to the body's hunger and satiety cues and relying on them to regulate the amount of food that is eaten. Conscious eating encompasses this as well as other conscious choices a person makes in order to create a diet that meets his or her individual needs and preferences.

As a conscious eater, Devon Kershaw does not simply eat what he always has or what the people around him do. Instead, he manipulates his diet in a variety of ways to make it work better for him as an athlete, a health seeker, and a person. In short, he is a role model for Habit 5 of the Endurance Diet—eating individually—and for its benefits: excellent health, maximum fitness, optimal performance, and great dietary satisfaction.

How to Eat Individually

Imagine you're standing on a vast grid that stretches almost infinitely in every direction. This grid represents all of the ways you could possibly eat—every collection of eating habits you might have. But you can't access the whole grid. You are surrounded on all four sides by barriers that keep you confined to one area. These barriers represent the first four habits of the Endurance Diet. Their function is to keep you from venturing into dietary territory that prevents athletes and exercisers from attaining maximum endurance fitness. Specifically, these barriers confine you to the part of the dietary grid that is defined by including all types of foods in the diet, eating mostly high-quality foods, placing carbohydrate-rich foods at the center of most meals and snacks, and relying on mindful attention to internal signals of hunger and satiety to control the amount of food you eat.

There is plenty of room to move around within this area of the dietary grid. The first four habits of the Endurance Diet do not force all athletes and exercisers to eat precisely the same types and amounts of food on exactly the same schedule. They allow a great degree of freedom to make individual choices. This is important, because the optimal diet for endurance fitness is unique to each individual athlete and exerciser. Somewhere inside the section of the dietary grid that is defined by the first four habits of the Endurance Diet is a specific point representing a version of this way of eating that is best for you and for no one else. The purpose of the fifth and final Endurance Diet habit— eating individually—is to help you find this point.

To be clear, the point on the dietary grid that represents your optimal diet is not a rigid set of extra rules that forces you to eat in precisely the same way every day. Your optimal diet still allows freedom to mix things up. Finding this point on the dietary grid is not about locking yourself into an inflexible daily eating routine for all of eternity but is rather about discovering and respecting individual needs and personal and cultural preferences that make you healthier, fitter, and happier as an eater than you would be if you passively allowed your circumstances to place you elsewhere within the space defined by the first four rules of the Endurance Diet.

In order to eat individually with success and discover your ideal version of the Endurance Diet, you need to eat consciously. Eating consciously comes naturally to elite endurance athletes like Devon Kershaw, but it's something that anyone can do. All it requires is that you make the choice to eat consciously today, make it again tomorrow, and so on.

Eating consciously means paying attention to yourself as an eater and acting upon what you learn. The final outcome of this process will be a customized version of the Endurance Diet that fits your needs and preferences. There are six basic aspects of diet in which individuality is manifest. To eat individually is to identify and accommodate your (1) needs and no-no's, (2) allergies and intolerances, (3) likes and dislikes, (4) cravings and crutches, (5) schedule and lifestyle, and (6) morals and values. Let's take a closer look at each of these aspects of eating individually.

Needs and No-No's

Scientists use the terms "metabolic profile" and "metabolic fingerprint" to refer to the totality of an individual's responses to diet. No two people have exactly the same metabolic profile. Genetic differences account for much of this diversity, but not all of it. Epigenetics (i.e., which genes are "turned on" and "turned off" in a person at any particular time), the microbiome, diet history, overall lifestyle, and psychology feed into the metabolic profile well.

Researchers working in the rapidly evolving fields of nutrigenomics and metabolomics are hopeful that their knowledge will eventually enable them to offer highly individualized dietary guidance based on each person's metabolic profile. Significant progress has already been made toward this goal. In 2013, for example, Harvard researchers discovered that a high-fat, low-calorie diet was more effective than a low-fat, low-calorie diet in the management of metabolic syndrome in obese men and women with a particular gene variant near the IRS-1 gene. Science is still a long way from being able to prescribe complete personalized diets for everyone, however, and many experts believe that it will never get there—that the metabolic fingerprint is just too complex.

In the meantime, eating consciously is very effective in determining which foods and eating patterns work especially well for an individual (needs) and which ones should be avoided (no-no's). A need is a particular eating pattern that produces positive results that are more difficult or even impossible to duplicate if that pattern is removed from the diet. A no-no is an eating pattern that clearly does not work for a person, even if it works just fine for others.

Devon Kershaw has discovered a number of personal dietary needs in his years as an elite cross-country skier. One of them came to his attention early in his career, when the Canadian ski team hired a young nutritionist with new ideas, one of which was to perform some workouts in a carbohydrate-fasted state (an advanced practice that I will discuss in detail in Chapter 9). Kershaw found that these sessions left him feeling run down and disrupted the flow of his training, so he gave them up. Ever since then, he has considered high-carb preworkout meals an inviolable need. But others, including Sara Renner, got good results from the carb-fasted workouts and kept doing them.

I define a dietary no-no as any food or eating pattern other than an allergy or intolerance that produces a negative effect in an individual. One of Kershaw's no-no's is heavy reliance on nutritional supplements. He discovered this limitation after he was persuaded to place himself on a sports nutrition company's full supplement regimen, which was extensive. It seemed as if he were consuming more capsules, tinctures, and powders than actual food. Soon Kershaw developed persistent stomach discomfort. At first he suspected that he had picked up some kind of virus in his extensive travels, but because there were no other symptoms, his suspicions were quickly redirected toward the supplements. Kershaw took himself off the regimen and the stomach discomfort went away. Later, he put himself back on vitamin D and fish oil with no ill effects.

As these examples show, applying dietary consciousness to the problem of identifying needs and no-no's is relatively simple. It does not require that you keep a log of everything you eat and drink or create spreadsheets correlating various foods and eating patterns with sleep quality, energy level, body weight, and other outcomes. It requires only self-awareness and perhaps a bit of experimentation.

When your health, fitness, or performance changes in either a good way (e.g., a really strong period of training) or a bad way (e.g., unexpected weight gain), look for possible dietary causes. If the change is negative, use common sense and the nutritional knowledge you've acquired to identify the eating pattern that seems most likely to be responsible. The first place to look is at recent changes in your diet. For example, maybe you acquired a habit of snacking on energy bars shortly before a period of unexpected weight gain began. Next, eliminate the pattern you've identified or substitute it with a sensible alternative. If your hunch proves wrong, try something else. (I'll say more about so-called elimination diets a little later.)

When a positive change occurs in your health, fitness, or performance, finding a possible dietary cause is not as urgent, but it is still worthwhile because knowing what works will help ensure that you keep doing it. In some cases, it won't hurt to try a small test to confirm your hunch about what's working. For example, if you notice that you perform best in your Saturday morning long bike rides after having a couple of glasses of wine on Friday night, there's no harm in not drinking wine the night before your next long ride to see what effect it has.

Alternatively, you may simply choose to believe that drinking an extra glass of wine on Friday night helps you ride better on Saturday morning. Such beliefs tend to be self-fulfilling. This is the well-known placebo effect. Psychology research has demonstrated that expecting positive outcomes tends to produce positive outcomes. Diet-based expectations for health, fitness, and performance are no exception. This was shown in a 2006 study in which recreational runners completed a 5K race 83 seconds faster on average after drinking superoxygenated water than they did after drinking ordinary tap water—except in both cases they drank ordinary tap water.

Marcel Holzherr has observed that many of the individual "needs" he accommodates when cooking for members of the Canadian ski team members are mere superstitions, yet he makes no attempt to break them. "It doesn't matter what it is," he told me. "It may just be something that's in their head. If they believe they will have an advantage, they will have an advantage."

Most needs and no-no's have a basis in physical reality and cannot be overcome through magical thinking. But it can be beneficial to identify certain "lucky foods" and other dietary needs that are psychological in nature. Many elite endurance athletes do.

Allergies and Intolerances

Allergies and intolerances are similar to no-no's. All three involve negative reactions to food. But allergies and intolerances are more specifically defined. A food allergy is an immune response to consuming a particular food that involves symptoms such as breathing difficulty and rash. A food intolerance is diagnosed when you have unusual difficulty digesting a particular food. It may involve an immune response but it does not result in the production of antibodies to the food as in food allergies.

If you have a severe food allergy, you probably know it already. That first trip to the emergency room after eating peanuts or shellfish (two of the most common food allergies) usually leads to a definitive diagnosis. Mild food allergies can be easy to miss, however.

Devon Kershaw learned that he was allergic to eggs six weeks before I met him in Canmore. He went in for allergy testing as part of a comprehensive effort to figure out why he'd had such a hard time shaking the illnesses that destroyed his 2014–2015 racing season and to ensure that nothing like it ever happened again. The likelihood that a food allergy contributed to his bouts of pneumonia and whooping cough was slim, but Kershaw was intent on leaving no stone unturned.

There is only one treatment for food allergies: the elimination diet. If the diagnosis is accurate, removal of the offending food from the diet will resolve the symptoms. The remarkable turnaround that American triathlete Amanda Stevens experienced after her numerous allergies were diagnosed (as described in Chapter 5) shows what a difference this simple treatment can make.

Note, however, that food allergy testing produces many false positives and false negatives, so you should have it done only if you strongly suspect you have an allergy and you should always let your body get the final say. Prior to his diagnosis, Kershaw had eaten eggs with vegetables every morning and never experienced noticeable allergy symptoms. Nevertheless, after his diagnosis, Kershaw eliminated eggs from his diet. He looked for changes in how he felt and functioned but observed none. Indeed, when I was with Kershaw he told me that he might eventually go back to eating eggs, which he sorely missed.

By far the most common food intolerance is lactose, which is not an actual food but rather a type of sugar in milk. Lactose intolerance occurs when the body stops producing enough of the lactase enzyme that is needed to digest lactose. Individuals with lactose intolerance often are able to consume fermented dairy products such as yogurt and kefir as well as hard cheeses without suffering the gastrointestinal discomfort that results from consuming other types of dairy. Because dairy is a high-quality food type with a unique nutritional profile, many lactose-intolerant elite athletes choose to continue to consume dairy foods that don't give them trouble.

The next most prevalent food intolerance is gluten, which, like lactose, is not a food but a nutrient; specifically, a protein that modern strains of wheat contain in large amounts and that some other grains contain in trace amounts. The majority of cases of gluten intolerance are self-diagnosed, but physicians do not recommend self-diagnosis of gluten intolerance because it is often inaccurate. In fact, researchers at Australia's Monash University found that only 8 percent of subjects with self-diagnosed gluten intolerance were in fact sensitive to gluten.

If you think you may have a food intolerance, make an appointment with a gastroenterologist and get a definitive diagnosis. Trying to do it yourself is likely to result in the unnecessary elimination of foods that are actually good for you. Also, although self-diagnosis of food intolerances tends to be inaccurate, the symptoms that cause people to make these diagnoses often are real. So by misdiagnosing the cause of your symptoms, you leave the true cause untreated. In the Monash University study I just cited, subjects who experienced no symptom relief when gluten was removed from the diet did feel better when foods containing low-fermentable, poorly absorbed, short-chain carbohydrates (or FODMAPs, a type of nutrient found in legumes, apples, cashews, and, yes, wheat) were removed instead.

Another problem with self-diagnosing food intolerances is that in many cases it exacerbates an already unhealthy personal food psychology. Studies by psychologists at the University of Birmingham and elsewhere have shown that men and especially women who self-diagnose food intolerances are more likely than the average person to exhibit neurotic symptoms, psychological distress, and severe depression. For such people, the perception that a food intolerance is to blame may function as an attempt to exert control over, and gain relief from, distress that is more psychic than physical in nature.

In my experience, perceived food intolerances seldom exist in a vacuum. Athletes who tell me they have one or more food intolerances usually also have a history of engaging in extreme dietary measures such as fad diets and purging. And despite—or rather, because of—all of the effort and anxiety they pour into "fixing" their diet, these athletes are seldom happy with any measure they try or with the outcomes.

Unfortunately, our society's current overhyping of food intolerances is expanding the pool of the susceptible. Food allergies and intolerances are real, but they're also trendy. Because dietary diversity is so important, I believe that athletes and exercisers should not avoid foods they need not avoid. So don't be too quick to decide you can't eat this or that. Try your best to tune out the hype, and when you suspect that you have a food allergy or intolerance, have it diagnosed and treated the right way, under a doctor's care.

Likes and Dislikes

People choose specific foods to eat for a variety of reasons. Research has shown that taste is often the most important consideration after price in food purchasing. In other words, people generally don't need to be told to eat food they like. But research has also shown that people whose main consideration in food purchasing is healthiness tend to care a lot less about whether food tastes good. This finding suggests that people are prone to assume that taste comes at the expense of healthiness in food and vice versa. Indeed, other studies have revealed that people give lower ratings on the taste of foods when they are labeled as healthy.

A tacit belief that taste and healthiness are mutually exclusive in food causes many people to subtly expect to derive less enjoyment from the experience of eating when they make efforts to eat healthier. This assumption may even cause people to make less of an effort to find and prepare healthy foods they actually do like than they would if they believed otherwise. Such resignation often dooms the healthier new diet to failure. Few people are able to sustain a diet they don't enjoy.

Elite endurance athletes enjoy their healthy diet because they allow themselves the freedom to choose foods they like and to avoid foods they don't like within the framework defined by their quality standards. You can see this sense of freedom in some of the odd choices they make. Devon Kershaw's meat-wrapped veggies at breakfast is a good example. Kershaw came up with this somewhat weird concoction because he was not willing to sacrifice healthiness for taste, but he is equally unwilling to sacrifice taste for healthiness.

When you modify your diet to raise your Diet Quality Score, consciously do it in ways that preserve or even enhance enjoyment. Many athletes need to eat more vegetables to raise their DQS to the level necessary to get the results they seek. But some athletes don't like vegetables. Or don't they? In fact, I've never met a self-professed vegetable hater who truly hated all vegetables. There are a million ways to add them to the diet. Don't force yourself to eat brussels sprouts if they make you gag. Instead choose vegetables and find ways of preparing them that you really like. A bowl of split pea soup counts as a vegetable serving in the DQS, and it's a lot tastier to some vegetable haters than brussels sprouts. If you need to add a little (unprocessed) meat to your pea soup or dip some (whole-grain) bread into it to make it acceptable to your palate, go right ahead. And if you don't like split pea soup, try lentil soup, baked sweet potato fries, a fruit smoothie with kale, or steamed broccoli with a bit of melted cheese. In short, don't give up!

My definition of "like" as it relates to food goes beyond taste to encompass comfort and familiarity. All too often, athletes and exercisers feel compelled to give up familiar and comforting foods that are perfectly healthy when they are seeking to improve their diet because of how these foods are perceived. I am often laughed at when I admit that I eat cereal and milk for breakfast. People think it's unhealthy. But I don't eat sugar-coated fruity bears or whatever the sweet cereal of the day is. I eat 100 percent whole-grain cereal with minimal added sugar, I pour organic whole milk on it, and I top it with fresh berries. That's 6 DQS points right there. Equally important, it's familiar (I've been eating it my whole life), it's comforting, and it tastes good to me.

You may be amazed by how much easier and more enjoyable it is to raise your diet quality standards if you simply give yourself permission to eat only foods you like and avoid foods you don't like.

Cravings and Crutches

Devon Kershaw doesn't have a lot of dietary rules, but among the few he does enforce is his Saturday Rule. Each week, Kershaw tries to make it until Saturday before he allows himself to eat one of his favorite low-quality food treats, such as *pain au chocolat*, a decadent pastry that he sometimes enjoys as a treat when traveling in Europe. He doesn't always make it, and when he doesn't make it he quickly forgives himself and moves on; but he always tries.

Most elite endurance athletes have rules—some explicit, others implicit— that govern their consumption of favorite low-quality food cravings and crutches. Although the specific rules vary from person to person, their underlying spirit and practical purpose are always the same. They serve to make athletes conscious of their low-quality food intake and to ensure that favorite treats are eaten often enough to keep them happy with their diet but not so often that they reduce the overall quality of the diet to unacceptable levels.

Another example of how elite endurance athletes use personal rules to control their intake of cravings and crutches came to me from Nuno Bico, a Portuguese professional cyclist. Bico told me that, during the competitive season, he drinks beer only after successful races and eats desserts only after especially hard training sessions. But in October and November he removes these restrictions and on Christmas and New Year's Eve he permits himself to get tipsy.

What makes such rules effective is their specificity. The frequency with which, or occasions on which, unhealthy food treats are allowed to be consumed is precisely defined. Too many recreational athletes and exercisers try to practice personal food rules that lack such specificity. Instead of allowing themselves to eat (or drink) cravings and crutches on specific occasions or with a specific frequency, they just try to generally avoid eating them—except when they feel like making a special exception.

The trouble with handling cravings and crutches as special exceptions is that most people have a remarkable ability to fool themselves about how often they actually give in to temptations. When people have specific rules for treats, they keep count. When treats are exceptions, people don't keep count and it becomes easy for them to convince themselves that they don't eat their favorite cravings and crutches as often as they actually do. A specific intention to eat potato chips (or whatever) once a week almost always yields better results than a vague intention not to eat potato chips very often.

This doesn't mean you need to keep a ledger in which you track your consumption of potato chips or bonbons or whatever your favorite low-quality food (or drink) happens to be. But what you should do is take a cue from elite endurance athletes and apply dietary consciousness to the regulation of treats in your diet. Decide on a frequency of treat consumption that is acceptable for you and be aware of how often you do in fact indulge in potato chips, bonbons, or fill-in-the-blank.

The best rules for cravings and crutches come from within—they are not copied from others. A rule that you generate for yourself is more likely to strike the right balance between strictness and permissiveness for you. Love ice cream? Have a small serving once a day, but make it the only sweet you allow yourself. Got a thing for beer? Choose one night each week on which to suspend your normal one-drink limit. Have a weakness for a certain fast-food burger? Reserve it for occasions when you've got something to celebrate.

The Diet Quality Score will help you keep such indulgences in check. If you're ever concerned about "indulgence creep" in your diet, calculate your DQS. Scores falling short of your target indicate that it's time to hold a firmer line on the low-quality foods you can't live without (and need not live without, provided you eat them consciously).

Schedule and Lifestyle

Some people love to cook and have time to cook often. Others don't. Some people have plenty of money to spend on food. Others have tight budgets. Some people travel frequently for work. Others wake up in the same bed every day. In short, different people have different schedules and lifestyles, and these differences affect their diet. Practicing the Endurance Diet habit of eating individually includes customizing your diet in ways that work with your schedule and lifestyle.

Elite endurance athletes tend to do this very well because, as with other components of dietary customization, they do it consciously. Devon Kershaw travels extensively for training and racing. Over the years he has acquired a variety of tricks that enable him to maintain high standards for diet quality despite the challenges that come with being in transit and in unfamiliar settings. For example, on flying days he packs his own fruit and vegetables and sometimes even a full meal instead of (as he puts it) "eating the junk you can buy at the airport or what they give you on planes."

Kershaw's lifestyle changed somewhat shortly before I met him, when he got engaged to Kristin Størmer Steira, a Norwegian elite cross-country skier who is now retired. Marriage and cohabitation almost always require dietary compromises, but oftentimes they create dietary opportunities as well. Like most Norwegians, Steira likes to eat fish. Kershaw embraced this preference and now eats fish three or four times a week. He has also added a few classically Norwegian foods to his diet, including the delectable brown cheese he shared with me.

Each person's schedule and lifestyle impose certain constraints on diet, cutting off some options and steering the person toward others. Nobody's schedule or lifestyle makes healthy eating impossible. With a conscious approach and a little common sense, it's not difficult to figure out how to make the Endurance Diet work in the specific context of any daily routine. Most of the challenges encountered in this process need to be solved only once and then they're solved for good—Devon Kershaw's trick for avoiding unhealthy airport and airplane food being one example.

Among the most common schedule and lifestyle constraints that make healthy eating a challenge are not liking to or having little time to cook, being on a tight budget, having a family, eating out often, traveling frequently, and having a hectic and/or erratic work schedule. Table 7.1 offers quick tips for working through each of these constraints.

Table 7.1 Tips for Working through Common Schedule/Lifestyle-Related Dietary Constraints

Constraint	Tips
Little time for or interest in cooking	Take advantage of healthy prepared and semiprepared foods such as microwavable brown rice and quinoa
	Try a service such as Blue Apron that will "hold your hand" through the cooking process
	Start with Georgie Fear's Level 1 Recipes in our *Racing Weight Cookbook*
Tight budget	Skip the organic produce but don't skip the produce (check out ewg.org's annual list of the Clean Fifteen and the Dirty Dozen)
	Start your own vegetable and herb garden
	Join a food co-op
Having a family	Start a list of healthy meals everyone likes and add to it one meal at a time
	Do little things to individualize shared meals, such as letting everyone else in the family put sauce over regular spaghetti while you have the whole wheat kind
	Make a family "game" of healthy eating, for example with the DQS app
Eating out often	"Collect" favorite restaurants with healthy menu items you like
	Pretend you're a vegetarian—often this will lead you to the healthiest options
	Before you go out, "spoil" your appetite a bit with a healthy snack and thereby lower your susceptibility to temptation and overeating
Traveling frequently	Identify the best options at even the worst places, such as 100 percent vegetable juice and dried fruit at convenience stores
	Identify the most reliable restaurant at each airport for healthy meals you like
	Practice Devon Kershaw's trick and bring food with you
	Pretend you're a vegetarian (see above)
Hectic/erratic work schedule	Keep healthy snacks such as fruit and nuts stashed at your workspace
	Organize your days into types and make a healthy eating plan for each type of day
	Find ways to keep mealtimes "sacred," for example by not scheduling meetings between 11:00 a.m. and 1:00 p.m.

Morals and Values

Would you eat your neighbor's cat? Probably not. Why not? Because it would go against your morals and values. Everyone's eating decisions are influenced by morals and values, whether this influence is recognized or not. Some people apply their sense of right and wrong very consciously in their food choices. It is not my place to tell you what your food-related morals and values should be, but I do encourage you to think about them when deciding which foods to buy and eat. It's one more way of making your diet truly yours.

Devon Kershaw purchases only seafood that bears Canada's Ocean Wise label, which indicates that the food is sustainably sourced. He told me, "Since fish is one of my favorite protein sources (and I love fishing!), I want us (humanity) to enjoy the seas', rivers', and lakes' bounty for generations. I think the best way a consumer can help is try when you can to purchase ethically caught seafood. Of course, sometimes you can't, but you can always try and I am cognizant of it."

Table 7.2 presents some of the most common value-based food choices and the advantages and disadvantages of each. Use it to organize your thoughts about how you wish to apply your morals and values to your food choices.

Table 7.2   Advantages and Disadvantage of Moral/Value-Based Dietary Choices

Choice	Advantage(s)	Disadvantage(s)
Eating organic foods	Encourages sustainable farming and animal husbandry; may result in a better-tasting and more nutritious diet	Higher cost; fewer choices
Eating locally grown and raised foods	Benefits the environment by eliminating long-distance food transport; supports local economies; adds fresher foods to the diet	Fewer choices, lack of access to out-of-season produce

Table 7.2 *Continued*

Choice	Advantage(s)	Disadvantage(s)
Avoiding plant foods from genetically modified seeds (GMOs)	Discourages food producers from pursuing a practice that may have negative unintended consequences	Discourages food producers from pursuing a practice that may have significant benefits, ranging from less world hunger to more nutritious fruits and vegetables
Avoiding foods that are unsustainably sourced	Discourages the fish industry and others from pursuing practices that could lead to species extinction and environmental degradation	Fewer choices
Avoiding foods produced with animal cruelty (e.g., veal, foie gras, but possibly also all forms of industrially produced meat)	Discourages the meat industry from practicing animal cruelty	Higher cost; fewer choices
Avoiding all foods sourced from animals (veganism)	Discourages animal captivity, cruelty, and slaughter; benefits the environment by reducing demand for resource-intensive foods	Less balanced diet

More Than Just a Solution

Every elite endurance athlete practices a unique version of the Endurance Diet. That's because no single set of specific eating habits is optimal for all athletes and exercisers. The four general habits of eating everything, eating quality, eating carb-centered, and eating enough are musts for every seeker of endurance fitness. But to attain maximum endurance fitness, each athlete and exerciser must practice the additional habit of eating individually—becoming a conscious eater for the sake of identifying and addressing personal needs and no-no's, allergies and intolerances, cravings and crutches, schedule and lifestyle constraints, likes and dislikes, and morals and values.

This won't happen overnight. It takes time to notice patterns of dietary cause and effect and to arrive at ideas about how to change eating patterns to better fit individual needs and preferences. Focus on the process of eating consciously rather than on the end point of the "perfect" diet for you. If you keep eating consciously, you will keep learning about yourself, and if you keep learning about yourself, you will keep moving closer to perfection.

You will never arrive there, however, because life doesn't stand still. The body is always changing, so what works for you at one point in life might not work at a later point. When he was younger, Devon Kershaw did not drink coffee, except before races, because caffeine is a proven performance enhancer. But he now drinks coffee every day. When I asked him why, he said, "I don't know. Maybe it's just because I'm getting older. I need a crutch." This might be true. Then again, it might not. Perhaps there's some scientific explanation. But the reason Kershaw needs coffee now doesn't matter. What matters is that he recognizes the need and knows he feels and functions better today as a coffee drinker.

Popular diets are typically presented as solutions—static and eternal. But the Endurance Diet, because it includes the habit of eating individually, is a solution that is also a journey.

8 Building Elite Eating Habits

Wᴵᴛʜɪɴ ᴛʜᴇ ᴘᴀsᴛ ᴛᴡᴇɴᴛʏ ʏᴇᴀʀs, ᴘsʏᴄʜᴏʟᴏɢɪsᴛs ᴀɴᴅ ɴᴇᴜʀᴏsᴄɪᴇɴᴛɪsᴛs have learned a lot about how habits and habit change work. Recent discoveries help clarify why some people succeed in changing habits—including diet habits—and others fail. Scientists now recognize that three special factors contribute to successful habit change. I like to call them *the power of reward, the conformity factor,* and *the principle of minimal disruption.* Although elite endurance athletes are no more likely than others are to be well versed in the latest science of habits, they nevertheless exploit all three of these factors to make the habits of the Endurance Diet stick—and so can you.

The *Merriam-Webster Medical Dictionary* defines a habit as "an acquired mode of behavior that has become nearly or completely involuntary." Habits can be as subtle and meaningless as picking at one's eyebrows while thinking (something I do) and as complex and important as performing heart bypass surgery with exactly the same procedure each time. We all know that habits are a big part of life, but we seldom appreciate just how big. It has been estimated that 40 percent of the actions the average person performs each day are habitual rather than products of a conscious decision.

The human brain is designed to form habits. It tries to turn everything we do more than once into a habit. The reason it does so is that habits foster both efficiency and proficiency. The first time you perform any novel action or behavior, you have to concentrate very hard on what you're doing. But the more you repeat it (the more habitual it becomes), the less active your brain is required to be in its performance. This process frees up your conscious mind to attend to other things. Without the ability to form habits, we would be extremely limited in terms of the number and variety of skills we could acquire.

A habit has three components: a trigger, a routine, and a reward. The routine is the behavior that constitutes the habit. Workouts, for example, are habits for endurance athletes. A trigger is a cue that causes a person to repeat a habitual behavior. An alarm clock sounding at 5:00 a.m. is the trigger that causes many swimmers and triathletes to drive to the local pool for a masters swim class. A reward is just that: some benefit that the habit confers, such as the feeling of accomplishment that comes with completing a workout.

The reason habits are hard to change is that they rewire the brain. Once a certain behavior has become habitual, its trigger compels us to repeat it, often unconsciously. At the same time, anticipation of the habit's reward creates a craving for it that is difficult to resist. A kind of psychological inertia develops, reinforcing the habit.

The neural imprint of each habit, eating habits not excepted, is essentially permanent. Once a behavior has been bundled together in the brain with a trigger and a reward, these three components of habit remain linked. This does not mean that habits cannot be broken, however. It just means that even after a habit has been broken, it remains latent inside the brain. This has been demonstrated in studies in which rats are taught one habit and then a second, contradictory habit in an effort to erase the first one. When these rats are reintroduced to the situation in which the original habit was learned, they don't have to learn it again from scratch but are able to revert to it right away. Other studies have shown that humans who have broken a certain habit are likely to revert to it under stress, again because its neural imprint is still present in the brain.

Eating is a special habit because it is an absolute necessity for life. Infants come into the world with built-in eating triggers (mainly the symptoms of physical hunger) and the act is intrinsically rewarding, offering the pleasures of taste and satiety. These biological exigencies ensure that everyone is in the habit of eating. Of course, individual persons have distinct eating habits. There is tremendous variety in what, when, where, and how people eat. But each person's eating patterns tend to be consistent. In other words, everyone's eating patterns are equally habitual. Like other habits, therefore, they exert an inertial force, resisting efforts to change them. Even so, people succeed every day in improving their eating habits. Understanding how they do will help you make a successful and lasting transition to the Endurance Diet.

The Power of Reward

We persist in our habits largely because we expect to be rewarded by them. Both parts of this formulation—expectation and reward—are important. What makes it so difficult for many of us to change our dietary habits is that, to a certain extent, this type of change entails shifting from a reward that is intrinsic to eating—the pleasure of low-quality foods—to a reward that is extrinsic to eating—better health, fitness, appearance, quality of life, and/or self-esteem.

The advantage that elite endurance athletes have in this regard is that they are more richly rewarded for improving their health and fitness than just about anyone else. Most elite athletes enjoy training more than they enjoy eating healthy. In other words, they are more intrinsically rewarded by working out than they are by maintaining their dietary standards. Nevertheless, they are just as disciplined in their eating as they are in their training because they know that healthy eating is as critical as training is to attaining the extrinsic rewards of money, fame, and the thrill of winning. Such rewards are out of reach for the vast majority of us, and that may be part of the reason our attempts to improve our diets more often fail.

This doesn't mean that, as a recreational endurance athlete, you cannot exploit the power of reward to find success with the Endurance Diet. The rewards of getting fitter and achieving goals are equally available to all endurance athletes. As the optimal diet for endurance fitness, the Endurance Diet yields these rewards in greater measure than other ways of eating do. What's more, the Endurance Diet can become habitual even before these rewards are experienced if you truly believe it is the optimal diet for endurance fitness and expect these rewards to come.

We touched on the power of expectations in Chapter 7. The importance of expectation as it relates to habit change cannot be over-stated. Psychology research has proven that if you expect to succeed in building new habits, including diet habits, you are more likely to suc-ceed. One example is a 2005 study done by doctors at the University of Minnesota. More than three hundred adults who had enrolled in a weight-loss program based on habit change were asked to rate their own chances of achieving their weight-loss goal. When the program ended eighteen months later, participants who expected to lose more weight were found to have shed the greatest number of pounds.

Expectations of success can come from a variety of sources. One is self-efficacy, or belief in your own ability to achieve a particular reward through habit change. Another is confidence in the method or pro-gram of habit change that you are using to pursue a reward. The more faith you have in the method or program you've chosen, the more likely you are to reap its rewards. But faith in a diet cannot be manu-factured out of thin air. We all need substantive reasons to believe it will work.

Elite athletes commit to the Endurance Diet because they believe in it—they have a high degree of confidence that it will yield the extrinsic rewards they seek to gain from it. And they believe in the Endurance Diet because they see what it has already done for other elite athletes. When a rising young elite endurance athlete looks around and sees that all of the top performers around him eat everything, eat quality, eat carb-centered, eat enough, and eat individually, it's natural for him to expect that he will benefit similarly from the same habits. A major objective of this book is to give you a vicarious version of this experience and thereby instill in you a similar expectation of success.

Obviously, believing in the Endurance Diet won't carry you very far if it doesn't work. But it really is the optimal diet for endurance fitness—and as such, it inevitably produces the expected rewards. These rewards complete the habit loop, creating a "craving" that impels you to persist in the five habits. When you get to this point, you're home free, because practicing the habits no longer requires effort. It is automatic, something you *want* to do.

What's more, there is evidence that healthy eating habits become more intrinsically rewarding after they have been sustained for a while. This means the longer you stay on the Endurance Diet, the less you will crave low-quality foods and the more you will enjoy and crave high-quality foods. A 2014 study led by Susan Roberts of Tufts University found that after six months on a healthy diet program, initially overweight individuals exhibited reduced activity in brain areas associated with craving when shown images of low-quality "calorie bombs" and heightened activity in the same areas when shown images of healthy foods of the kinds they were eating regularly on the diet (on which the subjects had lost 14.1 pounds on average). They were now as tempted by strawberries as they were by potato chips!

The Conformity Factor

Habits of all kinds, including food-related habits, are contagious. People tend to adopt the eating behaviors that are most pervasive in their social environment. Proof of this comes from a 2013 study conducted at Utrecht University in The Netherlands. Each participant was invited to choose a healthy snack or an unhealthy snack from a pair of displays. Empty wrappers were left near each display as evidence of choices made by previous participants. Sometimes the researchers left more empty wrappers near the healthy snack display; other times they left more near the unhealthy snack display. Subjects were found to be much more likely to choose the type of snack that appeared to have been chosen more often by those who came before.

These findings were reinforced by the results of a similar study done in the same year by scientists at the University of Birmingham. In this study, each subject ate a cafeteria meal with a partner who, unbeknownst to him or her, was working for the researchers. Sometimes the dining partner chose healthy foods, other times unhealthy foods. Again, the subjects exhibited a pattern of conformity in their food selections.

The good news we glean from these studies is that healthy eating habits are as contagious as unhealthy ones. The infectiousness of healthy eating habits works to the advantage of elite endurance athletes, who inhabit an environment where the five habits of the Endurance Diet are practiced almost universally. Being surrounded by men and women who eat everything, eat quality, eat carb-centered, eat enough, and eat individually makes it easy for each athlete to do the same. On the flipside, it makes it hard to do otherwise.

When I was in Spain with the LottoNL-Jumbo cycling team, I asked Marcel Hesseling, the team's nutritionist, what he would say to a team member who came back to the athletes' table at the Sala Oriente from the hotel buffet carrying a plate laden with French fries and pastries.

"I wouldn't say anything," he said. "I wouldn't have to."

What Hesseling meant was that the rider would feel so much tacit peer pressure from seeing the healthy plates of his surrounding teammates that he would never repeat his mistake. Indeed, the human propensity to conform to the dominant eating patterns in any given environment is so strong that no member of the LottoNL-Jumbo team or any other World Tour cycling team would dare to eat a plate of fried potatoes and cake in front of his teammates in the first place.

Most recreational endurance athletes and exercisers do not have the good fortune to eat routinely in the company of people who eat in the best possible way for endurance fitness. This disadvantage makes it somewhat harder for recreational athletes and exercisers to exploit the conformity factor. But there are things you can do to make dietary conformity work for you. One is to rally your family around the healthy habits you wish to sustain. Another is to share meals, recipes, and tips with training partners and other friends whom you regard as positive dietary influences. You can also use social media to your advantage, for example, by joining a Facebook group of like-minded eaters.

The Principle of Minimal Disruption

The principle of minimal disruption is the idea that, when changing a habit, you should change it as little as necessary in order to achieve the desired result. The reason is that it is easier to make small habit changes than it is to make drastic ones. This doesn't mean smokers are better off reducing their habit from one pack a day to half a pack instead of quitting completely. If a smoker's goal is to break the addiction, he or she cannot achieve it by merely smoking less. However, the person can still take advantage of the principle of minimal disruption by inserting a new behavior between an existing trigger and an existing reward.

In *The Power of Habit*, Charles Duhigg tells the story of a smoker who kicked the habit in precisely this way. He recognized that a feeling of restlessness was his trigger for lighting up and that a feeling of relaxation was one of its rewards. After trying a few different things, he settled on meditation as an alternative to smoking. Like smoking, meditation relaxed him, so it did not take him long to develop a craving to meditate rather than to smoke when he felt restless.

Changing eating habits is definitely different from giving up smoking, but not so drastically different. As I mentioned earlier, what makes it so hard for many people to change their dietary habits is that it entails shifting from a reward that is intrinsic to eating (pleasure) to a reward that is extrinsic to it (fitness). Many low-quality foods are more pleasurable to eat compared to most high-quality foods. Studies have even shown that processed calorie bombs alter brain chemistry in ways that enhance cravings for them, making them even harder to give up.

There is disagreement among scientists as to whether particular foods, or whether eating in general, is ever truly addictive in the same sense that drugs like nicotine are, but in any case the solution is the same. As with smoking, people are more likely to succeed in changing their eating habits if instead of simply saying "no" to their existing habits they say "yes" to alternative habits that address the same trigger (a craving for pleasurable food) and offer the same intrinsic reward (pleasure) but do so in a way that yields the extrinsic reward of fitness.

In addition to yielding better fitness than other diets, the Endurance Diet offers more intrinsic satisfaction than most popular diets because it is not drastically different from the way people naturally like to eat. In other words, it is less *disruptive* to normal ways of eating.

Most people—especially people with unhealthy diets—are comfortable with their current eating habits; they just don't like the results they're getting from them. Dietary change should aim to improve the results without sacrificing the comfort. The way to do this is to continue to eat as familiarly as possible while making changes that are sufficient to produce the desired results. The Endurance Diet allows and even encourages this.

If you look at what's on the breakfast, lunch, or dinner plate of an elite endurance athlete, as we have done throughout this book, you won't see anything that stands out as unusual or extreme except the overall quality of the food combinations. Switching from a merely average diet to the Endurance Diet is less disruptive, requiring less change, than shifting to the various popular diets that recreational endurance athletes often go for.

There is an inverse relationship between how abnormal a diet is and how long its average follower is able to stay on it. One of the most extreme diets is the raw food diet. A prominent apostate of this way of eating has estimated that 99 percent of people who try an all-raw diet eventually give it up. By contrast, elite athletes who adopt the Endurance Diet almost never quit.

Each of the five key habits contributes to the sustainability of the Endurance Diet as a whole. Eating everything is a natural human predilection. Eating quality creates a craving for quality, as was shown in the study by Susan Roberts described earlier. Eating carb-centered feels comfortable because most traditional cultural cuisines are carb-centered. Eating enough requires no more willpower than mindless overeating because it is not a denial of hunger (as in eating restraint) but an embrace of true physical hunger as the basis for decisions about when and how much to eat.

Eating individually contributes to the sustainability of the Endurance Diet in a different way. Although the first four habits make the diet generally comfortable for all athletes, the fifth habit makes the transition to it smooth and easy for each athlete separately. Eating individually is all about creating a personalized version of the diet that is based on a single athlete's needs and preferences.

When elite athletes transition to the diet, they do not toss out all of their existing dietary practices and replace them with a completely new set of practices borrowed from someone else. Instead they change as little as necessary to bring their diet up to Endurance Diet standards, retaining all of the familiar practices that are consistent with its requirements. In so doing, they exploit the principle of minimal disruption to activate the power of reward and the conformity factor. An improved diet is more rewarding when it retains features of a prior diet that, though needing improvement, was at least enjoyable. An improved diet is also easier to stick with when it does not unnecessarily abandon some of the cultural and familial traditions that the previous diet conformed to.

The American pro cyclist Larry Warbasse offers an interesting example of how elite endurance athletes use the principle of minimal disruption to ingrain the five key habits. A Michigan native with a Lebanese mother who loves to cook, Warbasse was raised on a healthy diet consisting largely of traditional Middle Eastern foods (lamb, pita bread, etc.). He did not live in a dietetic bubble, however. The family went out for fast food occasionally and Warbasse ate as much ice cream as the next American kid.

When he began to compete in Europe in his late teens, Warbasse learned about the importance of diet for fitness and performance and embarked on a period of experimentation that eventually brought him to the same place it leads every other elite endurance athlete. "I have found that a simple, healthy, nonrestrictive diet (eat junk occasionally if you want it, don't worry about whether something has gluten in it, don't worry about lactose, etc.), works the best for me," he told me via e-mail from his home in Nice, France.

Warbasse's preferred breakfast is oatmeal with coconut milk, honey, a fried egg and two egg whites, and a mug of coffee. His favorite lunch is basmati rice and an omelet with two eggs and two egg whites. He snacks on Greek yogurt, apples, and berries. A typical dinner comprises a salad of spinach and arugula, cherry tomatoes, green peppers, and an olive oil–based dressing; fish, chicken, turkey or (once or twice a week) beef; and one of the following starches: sweet potato, spelt pasta, buckwheat, or rice.

Warbasse practices all five Endurance Diet habits. The typical day's menu just described covers all six high-quality food types. Warbasse eats few low-quality foods except during the short off-season, but, he told me, "If I really want something, I will have it." His breakfast, lunch, dinner, and snacks are carbohydrate-centered. He also eats mindfully, eschewing eating restraint, because, as he put it, "I would rather eat too much and gain a bit of weight than be depleted and cracked." And he eats in ways that satisfy his individual needs, for example, by liberally salting his food to make up for the exceptionally large amounts of sodium he loses in sweat.

What is somewhat unusual about Warbasse is that, unlike most elite athletes, he did experiment with more extreme dietary measures before settling on the same five habits that work best for everyone. "I have tried avoiding all sorts of food in the past: gluten, milk, added sugar, high fructose corn syrup, etc.," he explained. "I really found that the more you avoid something, the more you want it. So now there isn't really much of anything I avoid; I just try to eat a simple, healthy diet." A diet that, importantly, is not so different from the one he enjoyed while growing up.

Warbasse discovered in a roundabout way that adhering to the principle of minimal disruption was the best way to develop habits that he could sustain consistently and indefinitely.

The Perfect Day

The five habits of the Endurance Diet are *daily* habits. To practice the habit of eating everything is to eat all six high-quality food types each day. To practice the habit of eating quality is to attain a high Diet Quality Score each day. To practice the habit of eating carb-centered is to eat carb-centered meals and snacks not once in a while but every day. To practice the habit of eating enough is to eat meals that are sized and timed in such a way that one is physically hungry when each meal starts and comfortably satisfied when the meal ends. To eat individually is to practice the first four daily habits in ways that meet individual needs and preferences.

If you can practice the Endurance Diet for just one day, you can practice it every day. Adopting the habits may seem daunting if you think of it as a matter of obeying a set of general rules for the rest of your life. But it won't seem daunting at all if you think of it as a matter of coming up with a workable daily eating routine that you simply repeat each day. Of course, this does not mean that you should eat exactly the same way every single day. But mapping out a single, optimal day's eating for yourself is a great way to get started. I call this exercise "the Perfect Day."

To begin the exercise, create a table with four columns, as in Table 8.1 (or use the blank table in Appendix A). The first column will be used to document your current routine. (Remember, adopting the Endurance Diet is not about *replacing* your current diet but evolving it.) Use this space to write down when and what you ate yesterday or, alternatively, when and what you eat in a typical day. Be fully honest and inclusive. If you spontaneously ate a handful of crackers yesterday afternoon when you opened up the pantry to look for something else, record it. We like to think of such behaviors as exceptions to our routine, but in almost every instance they are part of it. Include in this food journal some information about amounts, but don't be too fussy. For example, if you drank a glass of mango juice, write down "glass of mango juice" rather than "8.5 oz. mango juice."

When you've got everything written down, move to the next column and make a list of the ways in which your current routine falls short of Endurance Diet standards. This list should be fairly easy to compile, though it may require some review of the previous chapters.

For example, if your current diet includes no nuts, seeds, and healthy oils (failure to eat everything), note this. If your current diet includes more refined grains than whole grains (an opportunity to increase diet quality), write it down.

Now move to the third column and make a separate list of features of your diet that do *not* defy the five habits and that you'd like to (or must) retain as you move forward. This list may require a little more thought. If there are any specific high-quality foods that you want to continue to eat regularly—such as eggs for breakfast—add this feature to your list. Even if there are one or two low-quality foods—perhaps a second glass of wine after dinner—that you strongly prefer to afford a small place in your Perfect Day, add these as well.

Beyond specific foods, the list of current features of your diet that you wish to retain may also include such things as a preference to buy lunch on workdays at a great little deli located near your office, the need to stay within a very limited weekly food shopping budget, and a preference to cook dinners from scratch only on weekends. The Endurance Diet can be molded to work with most constraints, and you can always revisit them later if they become roadblocks to further progress in your health and fitness.

The fourth and last column is your Perfect Day. Here you will write out a specific one-day eating plan that evolves your current routine, as detailed in column one, by modifying it according to the information in column two and retaining the features in column three. This plan should include an approximate time for each meal and snack. Note that these times, as well as the number of snacks you eat and the amount of food you eat in each meal and snack, may need to be adjusted based on the results of the physical hunger experiment described in Chapter 6. For this reason, you may wish to complete that experiment before you create your Perfect Day.

There will necessarily be some arbitrariness in your food selections. For example, of the ten or twelve things you regularly eat for dinner that fit the design of your Perfect Day, you must choose one. But bear in mind that doing so does not fate you to eat this one meal every night for as long as you live. The Perfect Day is just an exercise to get you started on the Endurance Diet. Nor do you have to get it just right the first time. If, for example, you sketch out a provisional Perfect Day and then realize you accidentally left out the dairy category, go back and add it (removing one or more other items to "make room," if necessary).

As in column one, include basic information about food amounts but don't try to be too precise. If you need to eat a large bowl of oatmeal in the morning to stave off the return of physical hunger until lunch (or until your midmorning snack), write down "large bowl of oatmeal" rather than locking yourself into, say, "1 1/4 cups oatmeal." This information, alongside the schedule of meals, will set you up to successfully implement the habit of eating enough, but actually eating enough comes from listening to your body, not from executing a plan.

Use Table 8.1 to get a feel for the process, not as a blueprint for the actual content of your own Perfect Day. It does not come from an actual person but instead is based on a particular type of athlete I encounter often. Let's call her Brenda. She is a serious age-group triathlete who works out twice a day most days—early in the morning before work and again after work. She is concerned about maintaining a very lean body composition, and she does this currently by eating lots of fruits and vegetables, avoiding fat and starches, and limiting her portion sizes. If asked to name the biggest flaw in her diet, Brenda would point to her sweet tooth, which in a typical day she indulges with two diet sodas and a serving of low-fat frozen yogurt.

Measuring Brenda's diet against the standards of the Endurance Diet, however, reveals other flaws. The meals are too small for an athlete who trains as heavily as she does. The reason she snacks so frequently is that she becomes physically hungry well before lunchtime and dinnertime. To overcome this problem and find more energy for workouts, Brenda needs to let go of her eating restraint and start eating mindfully in order to eat enough. The specific energy source she is most lacking is nonsugar carbohydrate, so it makes sense for her to increase her meal sizes by adding whole-grain foods. Doing so will also raise her Diet Quality Score.

Brenda's current DQS is +5, which would probably strike her as surprisingly low if she were a real person. Although the large number of fruits and vegetables in her day give her a lot of points, most of them are taken away by the addition of sugar to her coffee (which makes it a sweet or low-quality beverage); her fruit-and-nut bar, which also counts as a sweet because it contains added sugar; the two diet sodas (low-quality beverages); the rice crackers (refined grain); and the frozen yogurt. Many athletes of Brenda's general type eat foods that aren't as healthy as they seem.

Table 8.1   An Example of a Perfect Day

Current Routine	Things to Improve	Features to Retain	Perfect Day
Breakfast (7:15 a.m.) Small bowl of low-fat Greek yogurt with blueberries and apple slices Coffee with sugar	Failure to eat enough (physical hunger returns <3 hours after meals)	Don't like to eat a lot of meat Like sweet things Breakfast and dinner times determined by workout times	**Preworkout (5:15 a.m.)** Banana
Snack (9:45 a.m.) Fruit-and-nut bar Diet soda	Not enough high-carb foods Need to replace refined grains with whole grains		**Breakfast (7:15 a.m.)** Bowl of oatmeal with blueberries and apple slices, honey Coffee with milk
Lunch (12:00 p.m.) Large garden salad Apple			**Snack (9:45 a.m.)** Mixed nuts and dried fruit
Snack (3:00 p.m.) Rice crackers with peanut butter	Too much diet soda		**Lunch (12:00 p.m.)** Large garden salad Whole wheat toast with cottage cheese Apple
Dinner (7:00 p.m.) Baked salmon Steamed broccoli Diet soda			**Snack (3:00 p.m.)** Carrot sticks with peanut butter
Snack (8:00 p.m.) Low-fat frozen yogurt			**Dinner (7:00 p.m.)** Baked salmon Chopped kale with brown rice Tart cherry juice
			Snack (8:00 p.m.) Frozen yogurt

Brenda's Perfect Day scores 25 DQS points. The big jump in quality is achieved by starting the day with a banana to fuel her morning
workout, adding whole grains (and replacing refined grains), eliminating one can of diet soda and replacing the other with tart cherry juice,
and upgrading her snacks. All of this can be done without leaving
Brenda's sweet tooth unsatisfied. There's still plenty of fruit, the honey
in her oatmeal gives her another little sweet fix and the tart cherry
juice yet another, and she still gets to end her day with frozen yogurt,
although the low-fat variety has been replaced with the less-processed
kind made with whole milk. Brenda may even find that her sweet
tooth is dulled somewhat by the extra calories she's getting throughout
the day.

The other items in Brenda's "Features to Retain" column are also
respected. She prefers to eat meat or seafood just once a day, and that's
plenty, so her Perfect Day includes no meat/seafood other than baked
salmon for dinner. Brenda might have addressed her hunger issue partly
by shifting the timing of her breakfast and dinner, but this wasn't an
option given her workout schedule, so the issue is addressed instead
in her Perfect Day through increases in the size of her meals and the
addition of a snack before her morning workout.

One Day at a Time

Once you have a Perfect Day you're satisfied with, consider creating
a second one. Some athletes need an alternative template for their
personal Endurance Diet because there are two different types of days
in their week. For example, a swimmer who travels frequently for business may need one Perfect Day for when she's at home and another for
when she's on the road. A runner who is divorced may need one Perfect Day for when he has the kids (who are fussy eaters) and another
for when his ex-wife has them. Many athletes need a different Perfect
Day for the weekend than they do for weekdays.

Whether you create one Perfect Day or two, here are some simple
ideas to keep in mind:

- **Practice makes habit.** Recognize that the purpose of the Perfect Day is not for it to be framed, hung on a wall, and admired. Its purpose is to be practiced. On the first day of your life on the Endurance Diet, try to apply your Perfect Day exactly as it is written. Pay special attention to your body's hunger and satiety signals and make any adjustments needed to ensure that you begin to feel physically hungry shortly before mealtimes and finish meals feeling comfortably satisfied.

- **Prioritize.** Don't feel ashamed of repeating your Perfect Day more or less exactly, day after day, in the beginning. Your top priority at this stage is to embed new habits, and the less day-to-day variation there is in your eating routine, the more quickly this process will move forward. In fact, there's nothing wrong with continuing to eat pretty much the same things indefinitely if doing so helps you stay on track. The diets of many elite endurance athletes are quite repetitious, and are no less healthy for it. A majority of the athletes who shared information about their diets with me for this book eat the same breakfast every day, and elite athletes in less developed countries eat pretty much the same breakfast, lunch, and dinner every day.

- **Mix it up.** A varied diet is optimal, though. You can add variety to your diet with little effort by making modular substitutions to your Perfect Day, replacing one type of vegetable, fruit, nut, seed, healthy oil, whole grain, dairy food, meat, or seafood with another. Further variety can come from cycling through the endurance superfoods presented in Chapter 10 and the Endurance Diet recipes in Chapter 11, and also from healthy recipes found in other sources. You can approach this expansionary process in a systematic way by trying one new recipe per week and by choosing one superfood per week that you do not normally eat and adding it to your routine.

- **Keep an eye on the big picture.** Never allow yourself to be tied down to your Perfect Day. None of its details are important. What is important on the Endurance Diet is that you consistently eat everything, eat quality, eat carb-centered, eat enough, and eat individually. The Perfect Day is nothing more than a tool that will help you gain momentum with these habits so that practicing them becomes automatic, something you do naturally without much thought.

Finally, always remember, too, that the habit of eating individually entails allowing your diet to evolve as your needs and preferences change, as they are sure to do to some degree. Adopting the Endurance Diet is about replacing bad habits with good ones. Living the Endurance Diet is about growing in good habits.

9 Fine-Tuning Your Endurance Diet

ELITE ENDURANCE ATHLETES TEND NOT TO FUSS OVER THE DETAILS OF THEIR diet. They focus on big-picture habits such as eating quality and spend little time and energy niggling over minutiae such as the number of grams of fiber they eat each day. The reason is that the details of diet don't matter very much. Or rather, the details do matter, but they are taken care of automatically through adherence to the Endurance Diet.

Consider the twenty-three essential nutrients (vitamins, minerals, amino acids, and essential fats) that we all must consume in adequate amounts in order to maintain our health. Getting enough of these nutrients is literally a matter of life and death. Yet with few exceptions (which I will address at the end of this chapter) there is no need to track their consumption, and the fittest and healthiest people rarely do. Simply maintaining a balanced, inclusive, high-quality diet will usually ensure that all essential nutrition requirements are met.

The opposite of the elites' big-picture approach to meeting their nutritional needs is what I call dietary micromanagement, which comprises an infinite variety of eating tips and tricks (or "hacks") that are propagated through popular media. Eat turmeric to elevate your mood. Eat lemon peels to improve digestion. Eat dandelion greens for better sleep. Although some of these measures may actually work, regulating your diet in this persnickety way makes eating unnecessarily complicated and is unlikely to result in better health. Dietary micromanagement techniques are clearly effective in drawing eyeballs to television and computer screens, but in the real world, the healthiest and fittest people, including elite endurance athletes, follow a few basic rules of eating and let the details take care of themselves.

There are, however, some exceptions to the elites' big-picture perspective on diet. Certain ways of manipulating diet that go beyond the five key habits of the Endurance Diet are proven to aid performance and are therefore widely practiced at the highest level of the various endurance disciplines. In this chapter I will discuss four such practices: nutrition periodization, fueling workouts, carb-fasted workouts, and supplementation.

Nutrition Periodization

The term "periodization" typically refers to the practice of dividing the training process into distinct phases, each phase responsible for adding another piece to the endurance fitness puzzle (a method we'll explore in Chapter 12). But an athlete's or exerciser's diet may also be periodized, and many elite endurance racers do eat somewhat differently at different times of the year.

As a general rule, it is best to eat consistently. The most erratic eaters are those who place unsustainably severe restrictions on their eating, resulting in a pattern of yo-yoing between superstrict and anything-goes eating. Elite athletes vary their diet in a different way, making minor adjustments based on where they are in the training process.

Typically, professional racers divide the year into two to three phases. Their baseline diet coincides with their major annual training cycle—the period that stretches between the start of formal preparation for the next big race or set of races and the last race of the competitive season. A shorter, secondary dietary phase immediately follows. In this "off-season" period, athletes may cut themselves some slack with their diet, indulging in a few more treats than normal. Between the end of this short phase and the start of the next training cycle, some elite athletes complete another brief dietary phase, a weight-loss focus phase, in which they set aside a few weeks to shed any excess body fat they may have accumulated during the off-season so they can then turn their focus back to eating for fitness and performance.

The Baseline Diet Phase

The goal of eating within a training cycle that culminates in a major race or a series of races is to maximize the fitness-boosting benefits of training. This is done through adherence to the five key habits of the Endurance Diet. The more careful you are in practicing these habits within this period, the better the results of your progressive training buildup will be.

Many nonathletes view exercise as a means to "get away with" showing less care with their diet. The more they work out, the more low-quality foods they can eat without consequences. But although this approach may work to some extent if your goal is to look good naked, it doesn't work if you're aiming at the higher standard of maximizing endurance fitness. When the goal is to get the greatest possible benefit from working out, then the period in which you are most serious about your training must coincide with the period in which you exhibit the greatest care with your diet.

Strict adherence to the five habits requires a certain level of motivation, but such motivation tends to come easily to athletes who are already highly motivated to perform well in races because they consider obedience to their dietary standards to be intrinsic to their sporting interests rather than separate from them. It is almost always easier to muster motivation for one thing than for two things.

This was shown in a study conducted by researchers at Stanford University School of Medicine and published in the *Annals of Behavioral Medicine* in 2013. The subjects were two hundred middle-age men and women with unhealthy diets who also did not exercise. They were divided into four groups. One group was coached to improve their diet and then, a few months later, guided through the process of starting a regular exercise program. A second group made the same changes but in the reverse order. A third group improved their diet and started exercising simultaneously. The remaining subjects comprised a control group that made no lifestyle changes.

At the end of the study period, the researchers assessed how well each subject was doing in meeting national guidelines for both diet and exercise. They discovered that those who improved their diet and started working out at the same time were most successful in meeting these guidelines. Subjects who started with exercise and then added dietary improvements later did not do quite as well in either category, but they did better than those who improved their diet first and started exercising later. And, not surprisingly, the controls had the worst results of all.

The researchers speculated that simultaneous diet and exercise changes produced the best results because subjects viewed them as a single project that drew upon a single pool of motivational resources. They hypothesized as well that taking up exercise first and improving the diet later yielded better results than the reverse because exercise makes people feel good about themselves in a way that makes them want to eat healthier. Elite Swedish marathon runner David Nilsson made this point in an answer to one of my survey questions. "The better your body functions," he wrote, "the better food you're craving to have."

There are both physiological and psychological reasons to maintain your highest dietary standards within race-focused training cycles. Doing so will give you the best possible results from your training and you will be most highly motivated to eat carefully at these times. If you're a noncompetitive exerciser who does not engage in race-focused training cycles, you'll want to follow the Endurance Diet as your baseline diet whenever building or maintaining endurance fitness is your top priority.

The Off-Season Diet Phase

"I eat less restricted in the winter," wrote Danish mountain biking champion Benjamin Justesen in response to my survey question, "Do you eat differently at different times of year?" Many other elite endurance athletes supplied essentially the same answer.

Like every other pattern that is common to the diets of elite endurance athletes, the pattern of allowing diet quality to drop slightly during the off-season period that follows the last race of the year is not arbitrary. It is practiced because it offers a benefit. In this case, the benefit is purely psychological. There is certainly no physiological rationale for indulging in eating more low-quality foods during the off-season, but it serves the purpose of rewarding athletes for training hard and eating carefully throughout the training cycle and replenishing their motivation to return to their baseline dietary standards when it's time to start the next training cycle.

There are some elite athletes who feel no temptation to eat more treats in the off-season, but those athletes who are so tempted find it easier to maintain their normal standards throughout the rest of the year when they allow themselves to lower them briefly after the big annual cycle concludes. It's like opening a valve to release built-up steam pressure.

Obviously, it's important not to go too far with this pressure release. If you lower your diet quality too much for too long you are likely to put on a significant amount of excess body fat and develop habit inertia around these "temporary" eating patterns that will make them difficult to break. I recommend that you limit your off-season diet phase to a maximum length of eight weeks. While allowing yourself to eat more low-quality foods during this phase, try to maintain the highest diet quality standards that still allow you to feel rewarded for "being good" during the recently completed training cycle and to replenish your motivation to start the next one. Continuing to monitor your DQS within this period will help you strike this balance.

If you feel a strong urge to eat a lot of junk during the off-season and/or you find it hard to return to your baseline diet at the start of the next training cycle, your baseline diet may be too restrictive. When practiced correctly, the Endurance Diet should be easy and enjoyable to stick to. A strong need to junk out for an extended period of time after the last race of the year indicates that you need to adjust the way you are implementing the diet so that it requires less willpower.

Nonathlete exercisers have no competitive off-season per se, but in most endurance sports the off-season coincides with the winter holidays. Many exercisers like to cut themselves a little slack with their diet between Thanksgiving and New Year's Day, right when athletes are enjoying a little break from hard training and racing. This practice offers the same psychological benefits for exercisers as it does for athletes, and the same guidelines and cautions apply.

The Weight-Loss Focus Phase

Many elite endurance athletes gain weight during the off-season. Putting on a few pounds of body fat is an almost unavoidable outcome of training less and eating less carefully. It's also not a problem. In fact, it's a sign that the off-season has served its purpose of allowing the body and the mind to regenerate.

Some elite racers do not gain weight easily and therefore do not put on much fat during the off-season. Many of these same men and women also lose weight easily through training. Athletes in this category typically transition straight from the off-season diet phase to the next training cycle and have no problem returning to their optimal racing weight in time for their first competition of the new season.

Other elite racers gain weight more easily and can't always rely on increased training to burn off body fat accumulated in the off-season. These athletes often insert a short weight-loss focus phase between the off-season phase and the training cycle. The purpose of this two- to eight-week period is to shed excess body fat faster than it is possible to do when training hard to attain maximum fitness.

As I first suggested in Chapter 6, the goal of maximizing fitness and the goal of maximizing fat loss are incompatible. The main reason is that the best way to maximize fat loss is to temporarily suspend Habit 4 of the Endurance Diet and eat less than enough to maximize the fitness benefits that result from training. This was demonstrated in a 2009 study led by William Lunn of Southern Connecticut State University. Competitive cyclists were asked to either reduce their calorie intake, add high-intensity intervals to their training, or do both of these things for several weeks. The cyclists who ate less lost body fat, regardless of whether they added intervals to their training. Those who added intervals to their training but did not eat less increased their power output. But the cyclists who reduced their calorie intake and added intervals to their training failed to increase their power output because their bodies lacked the fuel they needed to benefit from the high-intensity work they were doing. The take-home lesson is clear: keep your pursuit of maximum fat loss separate from your pursuit of maximum fitness and use the methods that are appropriate to each goal at the proper time.

If you are a competitive athlete, the best time to make weight loss your top priority is during the four- to eight-week period that immediately precedes the start of a race-focused training cycle. Consider engaging in a weight-loss focus phase if you are 10 or more pounds over your optimal racing weight at this point on the calendar. (Visit www.racingweight.com/rwe/index.html#/ to obtain an estimate of your optimal racing weight.) If you are a noncompetitive exerciser, you have more freedom to engage in a weight-loss focus phase whenever shedding body fat is your highest priority.

Eating enough is not the only Endurance Diet habit that should be temporarily suspended during a weight-loss focus phase. In addition to reducing your calorie intake, you should also increase your protein intake at such times, a practice that is, of course, at variance with Habit 3, eating carb-centered. You should also train differently during a weight-loss focus phase. Although a high-volume, mostly low-intensity training program and a minimalist approach to strength training work best for building endurance fitness, temporarily increasing the intensity of your cardio training and at the same time increasing the amount of strength training you do will help you shed more body fat when that's your main goal.

Reduced Calorie Intake

Aim for a daily energy deficit of 300 to 500 calories during your weight-loss focus phase. Research has shown that larger energy deficits produce less fat loss and more muscle loss. A moderate calorie reduction will enable you to preserve muscle while losing fat only. To create a daily energy deficit of 300 to 500 calories, you will need to estimate how many calories your body burns every 24 hours and count how many calories you're eating. There are a variety of smartphone apps that can be used to perform these calculations fairly easily.

Increased Protein Intake

In addition to eating less, reduce your carbohydrate consumption and increase your protein intake during this period. Aim to get as much as 30 percent of your total daily calories from protein. Although a high-protein diet inhibits the development of endurance fitness, developing endurance fitness is not your goal at this time. Your goal is maximizing fat loss, and increased protein intake aids the pursuit of this goal in two ways.

First, a high-protein diet reduces appetite, so that lowering your energy intake won't make you feel hungry all day. In a study performed at the University of Washington, overweight women whose protein intake was increased to 30 percent of total calories ate 441 fewer calories per day despite making no conscious effort to eat less, simply because the additional protein made them feel fuller. Increasing your protein intake to 30 percent of total calories therefore should make it easy for you to maintain a calorie deficit of 300 to 500 calories per day.

The second benefit of a higher protein intake during weight-loss focus phases is increased metabolism. This benefit was shown in a 2015 study published in the *American Journal of Clinical Nutrition*. For fifty-six days, male and female volunteers lived in a metabolic chamber that allowed researchers to measure their metabolic rate with extreme accuracy while the subjects ate different amounts of protein ranging from 5 to 25 percent of total calories. They found that the more protein the subjects ate, the more calories their bodies burned at rest.

Increased Training Intensity

Research has shown that the type of cardio exercise program that is most effective in shedding body fat is different from the one that is most effective in building endurance fitness. A high-volume program featuring relatively small amounts of work at high intensity works best to build fitness. I will describe this "80/20" approach more fully in Chapter 12. By contrast, a low-volume program with more work at high intensity is best for shedding body fat. So the training you do in a weight-loss focus phase should include fewer long-duration low-intensity workouts and more short, fast interval workouts than your normal training program does.

Increased Strength Training

It's advisable as well to place a heavier emphasis on strength training during weight-loss focus phases. Research has shown that men and women who combine a calorie deficit with strength training lose more fat and less muscle than do people who eat less without lifting weights. It's a good idea to strength train year-round, of course, but whereas two short gym sessions per week may be enough to keep you strong and injury-resistant at other times, three longer sessions will do more to help you get lean in a weight-loss focus phase.

The types of exercises you do should differ as well. Within the training cycle, you'll want to concentrate on doing functional exercises that help you perform sport-specific movements more effectively. I'll say more on this topic in Chapter 12. Within a weight-loss focus period, however, the emphasis should shift to exercises that build muscle mass, because muscle tissue burns a lot of calories.

Fueling Workouts

The purpose of eating (or more often drinking) while exercising is different from the purpose of eating regular meals. Breakfast, lunch, and dinner are intended to support overall health and fitness. Nutrition taken in during a workout or race is intended to enhance performance in that workout or race.

This distinction is important, because the healthiest foods to eat for breakfast, lunch, and dinner are not the most performance-enhancing things you can consume during exercise. Chicken and broccoli are healthy, but if you tried to eat them during exercise you might get sick to your stomach and you certainly wouldn't perform better. On the flipside, the most performance-enhancing thing you can consume during exercise is a sports drink, but if you routinely drank sports drinks for breakfast, lunch, and dinner, your health would take a hit.

The first nutritional product designed especially for consumption during exercise was Gatorade, the original sports drink, which hit the market in 1964. It had a clear purpose: to enhance endurance performance. Studies showed that it worked. The main ingredients in the original Gatorade were water, carbohydrates (specifically sugar), and electrolyte minerals. Each of these ingredients contributed to better endurance performance in a different way. Water did so by combating dehydration and by quenching thirst. Carbohydrates did so by providing an extra fuel source for muscle and nervous system activity. And electrolyte minerals did so by stimulating a higher drinking rate, hence further reducing dehydration.

More than fifty years after Gatorade's invention, its formula is largely unchanged. That's because no other nutrient besides water, carbohydrates, and electrolytes has been shown conclusively to enhance endurance performance when consumed during exercise, with the lone exception of caffeine. Nevertheless, many recreational endurance athletes and exercisers today avoid using sports drinks because they are perceived as unhealthy. But remember, they're not supposed to be healthy; they're supposed to enhance performance. If you consume such products during exercise and *only* during exercise, you will perform better and your health will not be compromised.

Following are some basic guidelines for nutrition during exercise.

Save It for When You Need It

It is not necessary to drink a sports drink during every workout. This practice can be reserved for challenging workouts in which you are pushing for a high level of performance. There is no need to consume a sports drink during, say, a 30-minute easy run or another low-intensity workout of moderate duration because maximum performance is not sought in these sessions. If thirst is an issue, you can just drink water.

Use Real Food When Practical

In workouts that last long enough for hunger to occur, it's best to rely on real foods such as bananas, trail mix, and biscuits, or on a mixture of real food and a sports drink, for needed energy. The reason is that you're actually missing meals in these multihour sessions, so the rule of eating for health applies even though you're on the move.

Drink by Thirst

Science has shown that the best way to regulate the amount of fluid you drink during exercise is, well, not scientific. Simply put: Your own sense of thirst should determine how much you drink. If you drink frequently enough and in sufficient quantities during exercise to keep your thirst at bay, you will perform better than if you drink less. Forcing yourself to drink more than you are thirsty for will not aid your performance but will increase the risk for gastrointestinal upset.

Follow the 60-Gram Rule

As for carbohydrates, the latest research indicates that optimal performance is attained at an intake rate of 60 to 80 grams per hour. It's less important to hit this mark in workouts than it is in races. Taking in even 30 grams per hour suffices to make a significant difference.

Simple sugars such as sucrose are better performance-enhancers than complex carbohydrates such as certain starches that are used in some sports drinks. The reason is that simple sugars reach the muscles and supply energy much faster. The idea that consuming simple sugars during exercise will lead to a "blood-sugar crash" and fatigue is a myth.

Keep It Simple

It's most convenient to get the water and the sugar you need to maximize your performance from a single source—namely, a sports drink. As mentioned above, these products also contain electrolytes, which stimulate a higher drinking rate and thereby further attenuate dehydration. Energy gels such as GU also contain sugar and electrolytes and are more portable than sports drinks, but if you rely on these products for your carbohydrate and electrolyte needs you'll need another source of water.

As with workouts, nutrition intake is not necessary during all races. Studies suggest that consuming fluid and carbohydrates enhances performance only in races lasting longer than about an hour. So don't be that guy or gal wearing a fluid belt in a 5K run!

Carb-Fasted Workouts

Within the past ten years, a growing number of elite endurance athletes have taken up the practice of withholding carbs both during and before select training sessions that are long enough or intense enough for carbs to positively affect performance. These so-called carb-fasted workouts are based on recent science showing that depriving the body of carbohydrates enhances certain fitness-boosting adaptations to training.

How Carb-Fasted Workouts Work

Consuming carbs before and during workouts enhances performance partly by allowing the muscles to conserve glycogen, their most precious and limited fuel source. If you've ever hit the wall in a workout or race, it was probably because the glycogen stores in your working muscles fell too low.

But something else happens when your glycogen stores become depleted: Your muscles respond by making new mitochondria, those little "aerobic factories" that use oxygen to release energy from metabolic fuels. And these new mitochondria enable you to go faster and farther before hitting the wall. So although consuming carbs before and during exercise enhances performance within workouts, it inhibits some of the fitness-boosting physiological adaptations that result from workouts.

This was shown in a 2013 study by scientists at the Swedish School of Sport and Health Sciences. Ten well-trained cyclists completed a 60-minute workout. Before the ride, half of the cyclists were fed low-carb meals and the other half ate normally. Measurements taken after the workout revealed that the gene responsible for creating new mitochondria had become more active in the carbohydrate-deprived subjects, whereas in the others it had not.

In theory, then, doing carb-fasted workouts with some regularity should improve fitness and performance relative to doing every workout in a high-glycogen state. Proof that it really does comes from a 2016 study conducted by researchers at the French National Institute of Sport (FNIS) and published in the respected journal *Medicine & Science in Sports & Exercise*. Twenty-one well-trained triathletes were separated into two groups. Both groups were placed on carb-centered diets that supplied 6 grams of carbohydrate per kilogram of body weight daily. But on four days each week, the members of one group got all of their carbs from their first two meals of the day and ate no carbs at dinner. These carb-free dinners followed an intense interval workout that members of the other group also performed.

The morning after the interval workout, all of the subjects completed an easy one-hour workout before breakfast. This workout was done in a mildly carbohydrate-deprived state by the triathletes who had followed the previous day's interval session with a normal dinner, but it was done in a severely carbohydrate-deprived state by those who had followed the same workout with a zero-carb dinner.

These dietary and training patterns were kept up for three weeks. All of the subjects completed performance tests before and after this twenty-one-day period. Members of the group that practiced carb-fasted training saw significant improvements in cycling efficiency, high-intensity cycling performance, and running performance within a triathlon time trial. There were no such improvements among members of the other group.

The purpose of this study was to determine whether carb-fasted workouts are effective, *not* to identify the most effective way to practice them. In the real world, no successful endurance athlete does high-intensity interval workouts on four consecutive days for three straight weeks, as the subjects of the FNIS study did. The most effective way to incorporate carb-fasted workouts into training is not yet known. In the meantime, it is sensible to emulate what seems to work best for elite athletes.

Practicing Carb-Fasted Workouts

One of the most sophisticated uses of carb-fasted workouts at the elite level is the system practiced by Trent Stellingwerff, a Canadian exercise physiologist and coach, who administers carb-fasted training with elite runners, including 2:10 marathoner Reed Coolsaet. Stellingwerff prescribes two to three such sessions per week during base training and one to two per week in peak training before a marathon. Some of these sessions consist of a long morning run at low intensity after an overnight fast. Others consist of a moderate-duration afternoon run following a high-intensity morning run and a low-carb lunch.

Other elite-level coaches and athletes do only low-intensity or high-intensity carb-fasted workouts, or do them with greater or lesser frequency, or do them only at certain times. In short, there is a degree of variety in how carb-fasted workouts are practiced at the highest level of endurance sports. Nevertheless, there are three general guidelines that we can draw from them collectively.

Make Sure You're Ready

Carb-fasted workouts are more stressful than normal workouts. Therefore, they should be viewed as an advanced training method and reserved for athletes and exercisers who already have a solid base of endurance fitness. You need not be a competitive athlete to benefit from them, however. There is evidence that adding carb-fasted workouts into a training program promotes fat loss, a major goal of many noncompetitive exercisers. Whether you race or not, though, allow yourself to get good and fit before you try carb-fasted training.

Ease into Them

Your first carb-fasted workout should not be a 100-mile bike ride begun on an empty stomach and fueled with water only. When incorporating this method into your routine, it's best to dip your toes in the water instead of diving in head first.

In the latter part of his professional triathlon career, former Ironman World Championship bike course record holder Torbjørn Sindballe of Denmark did what he called "zero-calorie rides." These bike rides were fueled with water alone but were preceded by a normal breakfast, so they weren't as challenging or stressful as true carb-fasted workouts. Sindballe's first zero-calorie ride was relatively short—1.5 hours—but as he adapted to them he was eventually able to go as long as five hours without hitting the wall.

Begin your foray into this territory in a similar way. Begin with a zero-calorie workout of low intensity and manageable duration or with an easier-than-normal high-intensity interval workout that is preceded by a low-carbohydrate meal or an overnight fast. If all goes well, do a slightly more challenging session next time. In the case of long, low-intensity workouts, incrementally increase their duration before switching over to true carb-fasted long workouts that are preceded by a low-carb meal or an overnight fast. In the case of high-intensity workouts, add extra intervals to them incrementally until they match the format of your normal, non-carbohydrate-deprived interval sessions.

Find Your System

Like other types of training, carb-fasted workouts will be most beneficial to you if they are incorporated into your training in a systematic way. But because the most effective way to practice this type of training is not yet known, you may have to experiment a little to find what works best for you.

There are three basic decisions to be made: (1) whether to do long, low-intensity carb-fasted workouts only, carb-fasted high-intensity interval workouts only, or both; (2) how often to do them; and (3) whether to do them early in the training cycle, late in the training cycle, or throughout the training cycle.

If you compete in long-distance events (e.g., marathons), you'll definitely want to do long, low-intensity carb-fasted workouts. If you compete in shorter events (e.g., 2,000-meter rowing races), you'll definitely want to do carb-fasted high-intensity interval workouts. And if your primary goal is fat loss, carb-fasted interval workouts are also the way to go. It is possible but not proven that the benefits of these two types of workouts are additive, and if they are you will get the most benefit from carb-fasted training if you do both.

Regarding frequency, although the FNIS study cited above showed benefits associated with four carb-fasted workouts per week, I recommend limiting their use to once or twice per week, for a couple of reasons. First, as mentioned, carb-fasted workouts are stressful. Work by David Nieman at Appalachian State University has shown that these sessions result in more inflammation than normal workouts. Also, performance is reduced in carb-fasted workouts relative to normal workouts, and it's important to do some—if not most—of your tougher training sessions in conditions that support maximum performance. For these reasons, carb-fasted workouts should not be overrelied upon. My own experimentation with carb-fasted workouts has shown clear benefits resulting from just one session per week. Two per week might be the sweet spot, balancing risks and benefits.

As for when to place them within the training cycle, I believe in sprinkling them throughout it. To use them early in the training cycle and phase them out is to risk undoing the benefits accrued from doing them previously. But to add them abruptly in the latter part of the training cycle may be risky in a different way, heaping a new stressor on the athlete just when he or she is training hardest. Gently introducing carb-fasted workouts early in the training cycle (provided the athlete has a solid base of fitness) and ratcheting them up from there minimizes both risks.

Supplementation

Elite endurance athletes are in a tricky position with respect to the use of nutritional supplements. On the one hand, they have a strong incentive to use any supplement that will aid their performance either directly or indirectly. On the other hand, they have to be very careful about what they put in their bodies. Many elite athletes who have never had any intention of violating antidoping rules have failed drug tests after taking supplements that they did not know were banned or that were tainted with banned substances unbeknownst to them.

Some elite athletes play it safe and take no supplements. Others choose their products carefully but never miss an opportunity to benefit from a safe and legal supplement that could improve their chances of winning. Most, however, opt for a middle ground, avoiding supplements that are purported to enhance endurance performance directly and instead limiting themselves to those that support basic health, confident that what's good for health is good for fitness and performance. A typical example is Ben Allen, an Australian off-road triathlete who placed sixth in the 2014 XTERRA World Championship. He takes iron, magnesium, a digestive enzyme, and vitamin C.

Even though most recreational endurance athletes and exercisers don't have to worry about failing tests for performance-enhancing drug use, I recommend that they take the same approach to supplementation that the majority of the pros do. The fact that very few elite athletes take supplements intended to directly enhance performance validates scientific evidence that there is no "must-have" supplement for endurance performance. Beta-alanine, sodium phosphate, and a couple of other supplements have been shown to boost performance in races lasting two or three minutes, but unless your event is the 800-meter run or the 200-meter butterfly, they won't help you. There is also some evidence that dietary nitrate and one or two other supplements may enhance performance in races lasting 20 to 60 minutes, but the benefit is minuscule at most and athletes can get it from natural foods such as beet juice (see Chapter 10).

Supplementation for health is another matter. There is solid evidence that some endurance athletes and exercisers may need to take a supplement in certain circumstances to avoid health issues that are pervasive within this population. Specifically, omega-3 fats, iron, and vitamin D are nutrients that endurance athletes and exercisers cannot always reliably obtain in adequate amounts by adhering to the Endurance Diet, not due to any failing of the diet itself but because omega-3 fats are rare even in high-quality foods, endurance training reduces iron absorption, and vitamin D is obtained mainly through sunlight, not food.

Omega-3 Essential Fatty Acids

According to the results of a 2014 study published in *Nutrition Journal*, the average American adult takes in 41 and 72 milligrams per day, respectively, of the omega-3 essential fatty acids EPA and DHA. That's bad news, because experts recommend that healthy adults take in at least 500 milligrams per day of EPA and DHA combined.

Omega-3 fats serve vital functions in the nervous system and cardiovascular system. Insufficient intake of these nutrients has been linked to depression, heart disease, cognitive decline, and other problems. In endurance athletes and exercisers, omega-3 deficiency harms performance in a variety of ways, including increased postexercise tissue inflammation.

Getting enough EPA and DHA in the diet is easy in principle. All it requires is that you eat oily fish such as mackerel, herring, sardines, lake trout, salmon, and albacore tuna two or more times per week. Even fish lovers don't always do so, however, and there is evidence that athletes may benefit from consuming higher amounts of EPA and DHA than they get from two or three servings of fish per week. For this reason, taking a daily fish oil supplement is advisable.

The benefits of doing so were demonstrated in a 2015 study by scientists at the University of Toronto. A mixed group of thirty male endurance athletes (rowers, runners, and triathletes) was given a fish oil supplement containing 375 milligrams of EPA and 510 milligrams of DHA or a placebo daily for three weeks. All of the subjects engaged in performance tests both before and after supplementation. Members of the fish oil group improved their performance in a standard test of anaerobic capacity by 5 percent compared to the placebo group and in a cycling time trial by 2 percent compared to this group.

If you decide to take a fish oil supplement, choose one that supplies the same combined amount of EPA and DHA—about 1,000 milligrams—as the one used in the study just described. Flaxseed oil and other plant sources of omega-3 fats are better than nothing, but their omega-3s come in the form of ALA, which is poorly converted to EPA and DHA in the body.

Iron

Iron deficiency is the most common nutrient deficiency in the world. The problem is especially common in poor populations, where red meat—the best source of dietary iron—is too expensive to be eaten often. But iron deficiency is even more common among highly trained endurance athletes, and in female runners most of all. Within this group, it is not diet but aerobic exercise itself that appears to be the main culprit.

Prolonged and intense aerobic exercise causes muscle damage followed by an inflammatory response that initiates the repair of damaged muscle tissues. Among the many biochemical changes that occur in the inflammatory state is an increased production of a protein called hepcidin, a regulator of iron metabolism. When hepcidin levels are high, dietary iron absorption in the intestine is impaired. Although research has shown that hepcidin levels are not chronically elevated in endurance athletes, the transient spikes in this protein that follow each workout appear to be sufficient to lower total iron absorption and cause clinical iron deficiency in many athletes.

When you think of iron deficiency in endurance athletes, you prob-ably think of anemia, a condition in which the blood lacks enough red blood cells to support normal functioning. Iron-deficiency anemia severely degrades aerobic capacity and endurance performance because red blood cells carry oxygen to the working muscles. But iron deficiency may have similar consequences even in the absence of anemia. That's because iron is not only a critical constituent of red blood cells, but it also plays a more direct role in aerobic metabolism within the mitochondria.

In a 2011 study, researchers at Cornell University investigated the link between iron deficiency and performance in rowers. One hundred and sixty-five female collegiate rowers were screened for their iron sta-tus. Of these athletes, sixteen were identified as anemic and another thirty as iron deficient without anemia. All of the rowers were asked to report their best 2-kilometer rowing time in the past three months. On average, the times of the nonanemic iron-deficient rowers were more than 20 seconds slower than those of their nondeficient peers. Although these results do not establish a causal link between iron defi-ciency and reduced endurance performance, they do establish a strong correlation that very likely indicates a causal connection.

The other headline from this study of female collegiate rowers is that nearly 28 percent of the subjects were iron deficient, either with or without anemia. The rate of iron deficiency is lower among male endurance athletes. This gender gap reflects a similar gap in the non-athletic population. Women are generally more likely than men to develop iron deficiency because menstrual blood loss increases their iron needs, yet women typically consume less iron than men do.

Female endurance athletes also eat less red meat than their sed-entary counterparts. A scientific survey conducted by researchers at Ball State University found that 40 percent of nationally competitive female runners avoided red meat "for health reasons." Another study by the same group showed that female endurance athletes who don't eat red meat had lower iron levels.

You can minimize your risk of developing iron deficiency by includ-ing a small amount of red meat in your diet and by regularly eating other iron-rich foods such as fortified whole-grain low-sugar breakfast cereals and teff (read more about teff in Chapter 10). Some athletes, however, become iron deficient despite being conscientious in their efforts to get enough iron through their diet. If you've been feeling a little sluggish lately in your training, the cause may be an iron deficiency with or without anemia and supplementation might be necessary.

Because iron is needed in small amounts (the recommended intake is 10 milligrams per day for adult males and 15 milligrams per day for premenopausal females) and is toxic in large amounts, I advise against taking iron supplements preventively. A 2010 study by Swiss scientists found that one in six male recreational runners exhibited signs of iron *overload* as a consequence of taking an iron supplement unnecessarily. It's best to have your iron level checked regularly (or whenever you experience unexplained, persistent fatigue and poor performance) by your physician and take an iron supplement under his or her supervision if your result is below normal.

Note that the best indicator of iron status in endurance athletes is ferritin, an iron storage protein. A standard blood panel does not include the ferritin level. You'll have to request it specially.

Vitamin D

Several years ago, my friend Reyana began to suspect she had iron-deficiency anemia. A serious runner, she felt lethargic during and between workouts and her times were slipping. But it turned out she was vitamin D deficient. Normal blood levels of vitamin D, or, more specifically, 25–hydroxy-vitamin D (25[OH]D), are between 40 and 70 nanograms per milliliter. Reyana's came back at 18 nanograms per milliliter—dangerously low. She was placed on a vitamin D supplement and after several weeks she felt like her normal self. A few weeks after that, she set a new personal best for the half marathon.

Vitamin D deficiency is easy to confuse with iron deficiency because both conditions cause fatigue and reduce aerobic capacity and endurance performance. The only difference is that iron deficiency causes fatigue by reducing the oxygen-carrying capacity of the blood, whereas vitamin D deficiency does so by reducing the capacity of mitochondria to use oxygen to release energy inside muscle cells. Below-normal levels of vitamin D in the body also hurt athletes by compromising bone health and the ability to manage inflammation. Additionally, there's a long list of health consequences associated with vitamin D deficiency, including increased risk for diabetes, heart disease, depression, and several types of cancer.

Unlike other vitamins, vitamin D is produced inside the body through exposure to sunlight. You might expect that endurance athletes who train outdoors get more than enough sun exposure to prevent deficiency, but this appears not to be the case. In 2012, researchers at the University of Wyoming reported that eight out of nineteen runners tested had "insufficient vitamin D status" and that two of these eight were outright deficient. Individuals with darker skin color and those who live at higher latitudes are most susceptible, the former because they produce less vitamin D and the latter because they get less sun exposure during the winter.

With very few exceptions, vitamin D does not occur naturally in food except in tiny amounts. Some foods, particularly milk, are fortified with vitamin D. Even so, it is difficult to obtain the recommended intake of 600 IU (international units) per day from the diet. Intakes as high as 1,400 IU have been shown to be perfectly safe. Regular vitamin D supplementation is therefore a good idea. Annual testing of vitamin D status by your physician is also recommended.

The most effective form of supplemental vitamin D is cholecalciferol. A daily dosage of 600 IU is plenty if you have fair skin, get lots of sun exposure, consume milk or other vitamin D fortified foods regularly, and/or have had your vitamin D level checked recently and are not deficient. Taking 1,000 IU daily may be preferable if you have darker skin and during the winter when the days are shorter and you're indoors more.

10 Endurance "Superfoods"

As a nutritionist, I've always been rather uncomfortable with the label "superfood" because it implies that the foods fortunate enough to carry it are somehow better than other natural foods, and that's just not true. *All* natural foods are super in one way or another. Indeed, a diet that was made up only of the medicinal foods like spirulina, green tea, and chia seeds that most often get the superfood label and excluded humdrum healthy staples such as oats and chicken would be incomplete and inadequate, especially for a hard-training endurance athlete.

Another way to define superfoods is to create a special category of specific foods that people with particular goals should try to include in their diet. By this definition, there are indeed such things as superfoods for endurance athletes and exercisers—or endurance superfoods.

In studying the diets of elite endurance athletes, I have noticed that the same foods keep appearing over and over, even in disconnected parts of the world. Like the five key habits of the Endurance Diet, this pattern is no coincidence. Certain specific foods fit especially well into the diets of men and women seeking maximum endurance fitness. These foods are characterized by a combination of tastiness, accessibility, familiarity, healthfulness, and, of course, favorable effects on endurance performance. Over time, elite athletes all over the world have identified the foods possessing this combination of qualities and incorporated them into their lifestyle. Whatever your fitness goals are, you will be well served to learn about these foods and consider eating any of them that you're not eating already.

Separate from the real-world process of trial and error through which elite athletes discovered these staple foods, scientists have studied the effects of certain foods on endurance performance. In some cases they have found clear benefits. As you might expect, there is a degree of overlap between these scientifically proven performance boosters and the foods commonly eaten by elite endurance athletes in far-flung parts of the world. These two overlapping groups of foods constitute what I call endurance superfoods. They are not foods that you absolutely must eat in order to achieve your goals, but they are foods that you are likely to find beneficial in the same ways the pros do.

Of the twenty-two endurance superfoods you'll discover in this chapter, only one of them—my wild card, teff—can be regarded as exotic. That's no accident. The virtue of the Endurance Diet is that it is practical, not radical or revolutionary. Part of what makes it practical, besides its beneficial effects on health and fitness, is that, in most cases, it is made up largely of everyday natural foods one can easily find, afford, prepare, and enjoy eating.

Don't forget, however, that the last of the five key habits of the Endurance Diet is eating individually. You shouldn't feel compelled to eat any endurance superfood you don't like or react well to. Few elites eat all of them. But there's no better foundation for your unique version of the Endurance Diet than the twenty-two foods highlighted in the following pages.

Almonds

Almonds have the same merits as other nuts and seeds. They are rich in unsaturated fats and plant sterols that promote favorable blood cholesterol profiles and healthy arteries and combat oxidative stress and inflammation.

Researchers at the Chinese National Institute of Sports Medicine have shown that these effects may enhance endurance performance alongside general health. In 2014, they recruited eight cyclists and two triathletes as subjects and fed half of them 75 grams of almonds per day for four weeks while the other half ate cookies containing an equal number of calories. After a two-week "washout" period, the treatments were reversed, with the former almond eaters getting cookies and the cookie eaters getting almonds.

All of the subjects performed 20-minute time trials on stationary bikes on three occasions: before the study began, after four weeks of eating almonds, and after four weeks of eating cookies. On average, the subjects covered 5.4 percent more distance in 20 minutes after the almond period than they did after the cookie period and covered 8.4 percent more distance than they did before the study began.

Try this: In addition to eating whole almonds and almond butter, use almond flour occasionally in breads, muffins, and pancakes.

Bananas

Bananas are among the most favored preexercise foods of elite endurance athletes because they are high in carbohydrates and easy to eat and digest. Even those who work out shortly after waking up usually find that they can nosh a banana before heading out the door without experiencing stomach discomfort during the workout. Serbian middle-distance runner Nemanja Cerovac, for example, noted in the questionnaire he completed for me that he always eats a banana with a little honey right before his morning run.

Because bananas come with their own natural wrapper, they are also one of the few natural foods that can be carried and consumed during extremely long workouts in which hunger is likely to occur. Daniela Ryf of the Czech Republic, the 2015 Ironman 70.3 world champion, has taken on-the-bike banana eating to the next level by scarfing chocolate-covered, salt-dipped frozen bananas during races. A 2014 study by researchers at Appalachian State University found that cyclists who consumed plain bananas during a 75-kilometer time trial performed no worse than they did when they used a sports drink.

Try this: Instead of tossing out those overripe bananas, use them in smoothies.

Beets

Beets contain large amount of betalains, a class of antioxidants with uniquely powerful anti-inflammatory properties, making beets a great food for postworkout recovery. Beet juice is even more beneficial for athletes. It has a high concentration of nitrates, which help the blood vessels dilate during exercise, increasing blood flow and oxygen supply to the muscles. In addition, they cause the mitochondria within muscle cells to generate energy more efficiently.

A number of studies have demonstrated that acute and chronic consumption of beet juice enhances endurance performance. In 2014, for example, researchers at the University of Cagliari found that swimmers were able to swim faster at a given level of oxygen consumption and consumed less oxygen at a given swim speed after consuming 500 milliliters of beet juice per day for six days. Australian professional cyclist Rachel Neylan is among the elite athletes included in my research who reported drinking beet juice before races.

Try this: When you buy fresh beets, don't throw out the greens. Although lacking the root's high concentration of nitrates, beet greens are rich in other nutrients, including iron, vitamin K, and beta-carotene. You can sauté them with garlic and olive oil as you would other greens, or pack them into a smoothie.

Black Beans

The many great endurance athletes produced by the nation of Brazil—including those whose diets were shared in Chapter 4—have been nourished and fueled largely by black beans, which are so important to the Brazilian diet that they have a category of their own in the government's official food pyramid. Research has shown that people who eat black beans frequently have an exceptionally healthy digestive tract. This effect is attributed to the food's "indigestible fraction," or its fiber and nonfiber constituents that pass through the body without being acted upon by digestive enzymes.

Try this: Mix cooked, mashed black beans with ground beef or turkey the next time you grill burgers.

Brown Rice

In most places where rice is a key staple food, elite endurance athletes still eat white rice rather than brown rice. But in North America and Europe, most professional racers have switched from the refined version to the whole version of this grain. Through their interactions with athletes and nutritionists from these places, Asian competitors are beginning to follow suit. For example, during one recent trip I sat down with Singaporean elite runner Ying Ren Mok to analyze his diet. Like many of his countrymen, he ate white rice at least once and often twice a day. However, I was able to persuade him to switch to brown rice. I can't take credit for the national record Mok set at the half-marathon distance a few months later, but the improved diet quality certainly didn't hurt him.

Both white rice and brown rice are good sources of carbohydrates, but brown rice has more fiber, protein, and phytonutrients and is associated with better health outcomes. A number of studies have shown that replacing white rice with brown rice in the diet lowers type 2 diabetes risk factors and promotes fat loss. Quinoa may be the trendier whole grain today in wealthy societies, but brown rice offers comparable nutrition and benefits at literally half the cost and is an easier switch for many rice lovers.

Try this: Order brown rice instead of white rice at Asian restaurants.

Cherries

Tart cherries have the most powerful anti-inflammatory effects of any food. These effects are mediated largely by anthocyanins, a type of antioxidant that tart cherries contain in high concentration. By controlling inflammation, cherries may accelerate postworkout recovery, increase overall training capacity, and enhance performance in races by reducing muscle pain.

Most of the research on these possible effects has involved tart cherry juice instead of whole tart cherries, because the juice contains a higher concentration of anti-inflammatory compounds. In a 2010 study published in the *Scandinavian Journal of Medicine and Science in Sports*, twenty recreational runners consumed either tart cherry juice or a placebo for five days before running a marathon, then again on race day, and for two days afterward as well. The runners who got the cherry juice exhibited less muscle damage immediately after the marathon. They also showed lower levels of inflammation and recovered their muscle strength significantly faster.

On a practical level, it doesn't really matter how quickly your muscles recover after a marathon. No matter what you eat or drink in the days following such a grueling event, you need to rest and then gradually ease back into training. But any factor that reduces muscle damage incurred during a race is also likely to enhance performance. Drinking cherry juice for several days before an event may get you to the finish line faster *and* get you out of bed a bit more comfortably the next morning.

There's also an argument to be made for drinking tart cherry juice during periods of intense training. In a 2014 study, sixteen trained cyclists were separated into two groups, one that consumed tart cherry concentrate for seven days and the other that got a placebo. Both groups trained normally through the first four days of the intervention and then completed a 69-minute ride at high intensity on each of the last three days. After the last of these hard workouts, the cyclists who'd gotten the tart cherry concentrate exhibited significantly lower levels of muscle damage and inflammation compared to their peers.

Try this: For dessert, heat some pitted cherries in a microwave until warm and top with a little ricotta cheese and almond slivers.

Coffee

Elite endurance athletes love their morning coffee largely for its caffeine content. A 2014 study revealed that 73 percent of more than twenty thousand urine samples taken from Olympic athletes over a five-year period contained traces of caffeine. The highest levels of caffeine use were found in cyclists, triathletes, and rowers. It's no mystery why. Not only does a well-brewed mug of high-quality coffee taste delicious and create feelings of well-being and mental alertness, but it also enhances endurance performance by acting on the brain to reduce perception of effort (i.e., make exercise feel easier). Other sources of caffeine, including caffeine pills, have the same effect, but the unique combination of caffeine and antioxidants in coffee makes it a multifaceted health booster as well as a performance enhancer. Regular coffee drinkers are known to be less likely to develop depression, type 2 diabetes, heart disease, and Alzheimer's disease.

Research indicates that it is safe to drink as much as four cups of coffee per day, but that's way more than you need to boost your workouts. I limit myself to one large mug in the morning to avoid becoming dependent on the stuff for wakefulness and alertness.

Try this: Drink cold-brewed coffee on hot days. A growing number of cold brew connoisseurs swear it's the way coffee was meant to be enjoyed.

Corn

Every culture has a favorite staple grain that serves as a major source of carbohydrate fuel for its elite endurance athletes. Corn (or maize) performs this function for the top racers in Central America, Kenya (the home of ugali), and a handful of other places. One cup of corn provides 123 grams of carbohydrate, along with sizable amounts of fiber, magnesium, vitamin B6, iron, and antioxidants such as lutein and ferulic acid.

Corn has acquired a negative reputation lately because in affluent nations all too much of it is consumed in processed forms such as corn syrup. But unprocessed forms of corn, including corn on the cob, whole cornmeal, and even nonmicrowave popcorn are true endurance superfoods. As with other grains, heirloom and landrace varieties of corn are the healthiest.

Try this: Use corn-based salsas on tacos and fish and in salads.

Eggs

Eggs are among the most ubiquitous foods in the diets of elite endurance athletes. I found them in the food journals of Brazilian swimmers, French stand-up paddle boarders, Russian triathletes, Japanese runners, and others. In a diet survey of ten professional triathletes from various countries conducted for active.com by retired pro triathlete Katya Meyers, nine said they included eggs in their breakfast either occasionally or routinely.

And why wouldn't they? Eggs are inexpensive, tasty, versatile, and nutritious, supplying 1 gram of high-quality protein per 11 calories, plus choline, phosphorous, vitamin B12, and other goodies. Once labeled unhealthy because of their high cholesterol content, eggs have been vindicated by recent science, which has shown that they are not linked to any unfavorable health outcomes.

Try this: Add thinly sliced hard-boiled eggs to green salads.

Garlic

A little garlic adds a lot of flavor to a wide variety of dishes. Science suggests it may also boost endurance fitness and performance.

In 2006, Japanese researchers subjected rats to a four-week endurance running program. Half of the rats were fed garlic extract before each workout and the others were not. When their training was complete, the researchers measured various biomarkers of fatigue in all of the rats. After analyzing the results, they concluded that garlic "ameliorates the various impairments associated with physical fatigue."

That's great news if you're a rat. But what if you're human? In 2015, Chris Womack and colleagues at James Madison University subjected eighteen healthy male college students to a graded exercise test after half of them had consumed garlic extract and the other half a placebo. Fourteen days later, the test was repeated, but the treatments were reversed. On average, the subjects' VO_2max scores were 2.7 percent higher in the garlic trial.

It should be noted that both of these studies involved garlic extract, not the whole garlic we cook with, and that other studies have failed to show positive effects of garlic supplementation on human endurance performance. So you shouldn't expect cooking with garlic to lead to major performance breakthroughs. But this can be said of any endurance superfood. Performance breakthroughs happen through the cumulative effect of eating lots of different foods like garlic that make small contributions to endurance fitness.

Try this: Who says you can only eat garlic bread at Italian restaurants? Make your own at home (using whole-grain bread, of course!).

Olive Oil

Of all the foods that the Sky professional cycling team might have lent their brand to, they chose olive oil. The decision to create Team Sky Extra-Virgin Olive Oil was not arbitrary. The members of Team Sky consume great quantities of olive oil and their coaches and nutritionists believe very strongly in its benefits for endurance athletes. And they're hardly alone. Elite endurance athletes all over the world consider it a vital component of their diet.

Olive oil offers several benefits to endurance athletes and exercisers. Antioxidant compounds in olive oil, especially hydroxytyrosol, prevent oxidative damage to blood vessel walls and other tissues. Other antioxidants, including oleocanthal, fight inflammation through a mechanism of action similar to that of ibuprofen. Olive oil also aids in converting cholesterol into testosterone, which in turn facilitates muscular adaptations to training. Finally, olive oil acts upon the neuromuscular system in ways that support endurance fitness. An intriguing 2012 study by scientists at the University of Florence found that supplementation with extra-virgin olive oil reduced age-related declines in motor coordination in rats.

All in all, the benefits of olive oil for endurance athletes and exercisers are as diverse as its uses in cooking.

Try this: Use an olive oil mister instead of olive oil cooking sprays (which are not pure olive oil).

Peanut Butter

When I visited with the LottoNL-Jumbo cycling team in Spain, I was struck by the vast quantities of peanut butter that Laurens ten Dam ate. But I wasn't shocked. Many elite endurance athletes rely on old-fashioned peanut butter (just peanuts and salt, no sugar or added oils) as a source of easy, high-quality calories during periods of heavy training. Too often dismissed as kids' food, sugar-free peanut butter is as wholesome as the peanuts it's made from and as nutritious as more expensive alternatives such as cashew butter. Indeed, peanut butter is actually higher than cashew butter in protein, fiber, and unsaturated fat.

Sometimes, when you're training hard, you need a go-to comfort food that you can use to quickly fill the void without sacrificing your quality standards or breaking the bank when you eat it often. Peanut butter—spread on toasted whole-grain bread, smeared on celery sticks, or added to smoothies—is that kind of food for lots of athletes.

Try this: Use peanut butter in smoothies (it goes well with bananas, spinach, milk or yogurt, and honey, among other things).

Potatoes

In his memoir *Running to the Top*, Australia's Derek Clayton, who set marathon world records in 1967 and 1969, wrote of his diet, "Potatoes were so high as a source of carbs, as well as being efficient as fuel, that I found myself eating enormous quantities of them throughout my competitive career." Clayton is not the only elite endurance athlete who has depended on potatoes as an efficient fuel source. Alongside grains such as rice and corn, spuds are among the most popular high-carb staples in the diets of top racers in many parts of the world.

Anticarb propaganda has turned many health-conscious eaters outside the ranks of elite endurance athletes away from potatoes, but without justification. Potatoes are as healthy as any other natural food. In fact, they may be healthier than most. According to Adam Drewnowski of the Center for Public Health Nutrition at the University of Washington, potatoes provide more total nutrition per unit cost than any other food except sweet potatoes.

Other research has revealed that nonfried potatoes are one of the most satiating foods available. When people eat potatoes they get full on fewer calories and eat less in their next meal than they do when they eat any other food. So it's not surprising that, as I mentioned in Chapter 4, a 2014 study published in the *Journal of the American College of Nutrition* reported that the addition of nonfried potatoes to the diet facilitated weight loss.

From a culinary standpoint, the best thing about potatoes is their versatility. There are dozens of ways to prepare them, and they can be included in every meal. But some ways of preparing them—particularly deep frying—turn them into a low-quality food, so save French fries for special occasions. Sautéing potatoes in olive oil is okay.

Try this: Have a healthy stuffed baked potato as a meal every now and then. Topping ideas include chili with sour cream and cottage cheese with grilled vegetables.

Red Wine

After he won his first Tour de France title in 2013, Chris Froome surprised some people by telling a reporter for *The Daily Mail*, "Actually, on quite a regular basis we do have a glass of red [wine], even on the Tour. If we had a good day's racing, or even a bad day's racing, and the guys just wanted to unwind, we'd crack open a bottle. I don't think a glass of red would really do any damage and would probably do just the opposite, and help you to relax and unwind before the next day."

Many, if not most, elite endurance athletes consume alcohol in moderation for the same reason. Apart from its beneficial effects on the cardiovascular system, a nice drink does indeed help an athlete relax, and a relaxed athlete performs better.

The preferred drink among elite endurance athletes is red wine, and that is because of its beneficial effects on the cardiovascular system. All alcoholic beverages are healthy in modest amounts, but red wine appears to be the healthiest. What makes it special is resveratrol, an antioxidant that improves cardiovascular health by increasing the elasticity of blood vessels, increasing HDL cholesterol, and reducing blood clotting. In nonathletes, these effects help prevent cardiovascular disease. In endurance athletes and exercisers, they strengthen a physiological system that is vital to aerobic performance.

Try this: Join a wine club. This can be a great way to make wine exploration a part of your lifestyle without investing a lot of time and energy into it.

Salmon

In 2013, when I asked American professional triathlete Meredith Kessler to describe her typical dinner, she said, "We eat a lot of salmon in our household. My husband makes a mean miso marinade and grills the salmon on cedar planks, which tastes amazing."

This answer was not unexpected. Salmon has appeared more often than any other fish in the elite endurance athlete food journals I've reviewed. Its worldwide popularity stems not only from its much touted health benefits but also from its appealing taste and texture. Even many people who claim not to like fish like salmon.

Salmon is one of the best sources of the omega-3 fatty acids EPA and DHA. A typical four-ounce serving contains a combined four grams of these essential fats. Eat it twice and you've met your omega-3 requirement for a week. Less appreciated is salmon's high content of bioactive peptides, which are protein fractions that combat inflammation and oxidative stress. The fish is also rich in a long list of vitamins and minerals.

Try this: Eat smoked salmon (lox) with cream cheese, red onion, and capers on a whole grain bagel once a week or so.

Spinach

Spinach is perhaps the most versatile leafy vegetable. I've seen elite endurance athletes eat it raw in salads, steamed or boiled as a side dish to hot meals, and blended into smoothies. It is also one of the most nutritionally complete foods on Earth. Loaded with vitamins A, C, and K, a variety of minerals, and an array of phytonutrients, spinach earns a Completeness Score of 91 from Nutrition Data (a measure of how complete a food is with respect to twenty-three nutrients). That's six points higher than the green-of-the-moment, kale.

Of particular interest to endurance athletes, spinach is one of the best food sources of dietary nitrate next to beets. Recall that nitrate enhances endurance performance by increasing blood flow to the muscles and by helping mitochondria, the aerobic factories within cells, function more efficiently.

Try this: Add spinach to meatloaves, lasagnas, pizzas, and other comfort foods to make them more nutritious but no less comforting.

Sweet Potatoes

More than almost any other food, sweet potatoes are gaining new fans among elite endurance athletes. In the case of American professional cyclist Ally Stacher, the discovery of the colorful root vegetable's virtues made such an impact that she developed her own sweet potato–based energy bar (Ally's Bar).

Sweet potatoes are becoming increasingly popular among pro racers in large part because they are nutritionally well-rounded compared to some other high-carb foods. One cup of cooked sweet potato supplies 41 grams of carbs. But sweet potatoes are also rich in vitamins A and C, fiber, and the antioxidant beta-carotene. Their Nutrition Data Completeness Score of 65 is about 20 points higher than that of any whole grain.

Try this: Put your blender to work to make quick-and-easy sweet potato soups. Just bake the sweet potatoes until soft, combine them with your other ingredients in the blender, and press a button!

Tea

In places where coffee is less popular among elite endurance athletes—places like England and India—its cousin tea is more popular. It carries the same benefits for health and endurance performance as coffee. A 2013 scientific review conducted by researchers at the University of Wisconsin reported that green and black tea may reduce the risk of some cancers, cardiovascular disease, and type 2 diabetes and may also slow some aspects of the aging process. These effects are attributed to its caffeine content and its high concentration of antioxidants, particularly polyphenols. There is evidence as well that green tea improves brain function and reduces body fat slightly.

Despite its caffeine content, tea has been shown to hydrate about as well as plain water. Among Kenya's elite runners, tea is the primary source of hydration. As described in Chapter 5, they like to take it with plenty of milk and sugar. In this form it makes an especially good postexercise recovery beverage, providing water for rehydration, carbohydrates for muscle refueling, protein for muscle rebuilding, and antioxidants to combat oxidative stress. (Do take it easy on the sugar, though!)

Try this: If you're normally a coffee drinker, replace your morning joe with a cup of black or green tea once a week or so for a little nutritional and flavor diversity.

Teff

What ugali is to the cuisine of Kenya, the world's greatest running nation, injera is to the cuisine of Ethiopia, the world's second-greatest running nation. If you have ever eaten at an Ethiopian restaurant, you've eaten injera, a spongy bread that is torn into small pieces and used to wrap bite-size portions of vegetables, beans, stewed meat, and other delights.

Injera is made from teff, a millet-like grain that contains 50 percent more iron than whole wheat. A 2014 study by the Ethiopian Public

Health Institute found that only 2 out of 101 elite Ethiopian runners tested was iron deficient. Because Ethiopians eat very little red meat, it is likely that teff is responsible for the low rate of iron deficiency among the nation's hardest-training athletes.

You don't have to be Ethiopian to benefit from teff. In another 2014 study, researchers at Manchester Metropolitan University added teff to the diets of eleven recreational female runners from England. Initial testing determined that they were not consuming iron in adequate amounts. Their average intake was 10.7 milligrams per day, well below the recommended intake of 15 milligrams per day for premenopausal women. Four of the women also tested as iron deficient.

The runners were then asked to replace the bread they normally ate with bread made from teff flour. This one simple substitution elevated the subjects' average daily iron intake to 18.5 milligrams. This increase was associated with significantly improved iron supply to body tissues.

If you're concerned about iron deficiency, and you'd rather get additional iron from a source other than red meat and supplements, consider incorporating teff into your diet.

Try this: Start your day with a bowl of teff porridge. Toast the teff in a heavy sauce pan on medium-low heat before adding 1.5 cups of water for every half cup of teff and boiling until it's thick. Add whatever you like for flavor, texture, and extra nutrition: dried or fresh fruit, seasonings, butter or milk, and/or chopped nuts.

Tomatoes

Members of the Torque Konya Sekerspor Club pro cycling team from Turkey often include sliced tomatoes and cucumbers in their breakfast—but only during the summer, when they're in season. The Turks are particular about their tomatoes. Indeed, they are the world's ultimate tomato connoisseurs, consuming more tomatoes than people in any other country.

Turkish professional racers are not the only ones who take advantage of the food's special benefits, though. Elite endurance athletes in many parts of the world consume tomatoes frequently and in a great variety of forms—fresh, juiced, and in sauces, salsas, and soups. One of the great virtues of tomatoes is that they offer a lot of flavor and satisfaction without a lot of calories. (One medium tomato contains 22 calories.) They are rich in vitamins A and C as well as in the antioxidants beta-carotene and lycopene.

Among the special benefits of tomato consumption for endurance athletes is improved muscle recovery. In 2012, researchers at Stockholm University reported that tomato juice significantly reduced oxidative stress after exercise in a group of nonathletes. A year later, a team of Greek scientists recruited fifteen endurance athletes as subjects and asked nine of them to replace their regular sports drink with tomato juice during and after training for a period of two months. The researchers reported that the tomato juice drinkers exhibited significantly reduced biomarkers of muscle damage and inflammation.

Tomatoes are also known to improve the elasticity of blood vessels. In nonexercisers, this effect reduces the risk of cardiovascular disease. In endurance athletes, it enhances cardiovascular performance. This was shown in another study conducted by Greek researchers. In this experiment, thirty ultrarunners were given either a whey protein bar to eat or tomato juice to drink daily for two months while they continued with their normal training. At the end of this intervention, blood vessel elasticity was improved only in the runners who drank tomato juice.

Try this: Grow your own heirloom tomatoes. They won't keep you "in the red" year-round, but throughout the summer you'll be spoiled with fresher, tastier, and more nutritious tomatoes than you can get anywhere else.

Tuna

The award for the most interesting use of tuna I witnessed in researching this book goes to Canadian elite cross-country skier Devon Kershaw, who placed a dollop of Thai spice tuna atop a salad of mixed greens, kale, beetroot, red and yellow peppers, apple slices, avocado, olive oil, balsamic vinegar, and cottage cheese. Like many other endurance superfoods, tuna has the quality of versatility. You can sear a tuna steak in slices or whole, create a tuna salad for sandwiches, enjoy it in sushi, and even spread tuna pâté on crackers.

Another benefit of tuna is its healthfulness. That's why many of Devon Kershaw's elite peers also eat tuna regularly. It is an excellent source of unsaturated fats, which support brain function and create healthy cell membranes. Tuna is also one of the best food sources of selenium, a mineral with antioxidant properties. Scientists discovered recently that much of the selenium in tuna occurs in the especially potent form of selenoneine.

Try this: Replace mayonnaise with avocado in your tuna salad for a healthier sandwich that still tastes good.

Yogurt

Lina Augaitis, who won the 2014 stand-up paddle boarding world championship for Canada, starts each day with one of three breakfasts. Some days it's a smoothie, other days eggs and potatoes, and still others a bowl of homemade granola with fruit, almond milk, and yogurt.

I've lost count of the number of regular yogurt eaters I've encountered within the ranks of elite endurance athletes. Many of them like to eat yogurt for recovery after workouts because its balance of carbohydrates, fat, and protein is ideal for that purpose. But perhaps the greatest benefit of yogurt for endurance athletes is its effect on body composition. No fewer than three of its ingredients help athletes shed excess body fat. Protein promotes satiety, probiotics such as lactobacillus shift the balance of gut bacteria to reduce dietary fat absorption, and calcium reduces body fat levels through several different mechanisms.

Not all yogurts are equal, however. The healthiest ones are those without added sugar or reduced fat content. Many people assume that full-fat dairy products of all kinds are less healthy, but they are more natural (i.e., less processed) than their low-fat counterparts, so it's not surprising that studies have linked them to better health outcomes.

Try this: Eat yogurt with fruit and nuts after some of your workouts. It's a great recovery snack, not only for its nutritional composition but because it's easy to prepare and eat when you're fatigued from hard training.

11   Endurance Diet Recipes

IF, STARTING TOMORROW, YOU WERE TO EAT NOTHING ELSE BESIDES THE recipes presented in this chapter, you would be on the Endurance Diet. The habits of eating everything, eating quality, and eating carb-centered are built into the recipes. All that's left for you to do is eat enough of them by eating mindfully and to tailor them to your individual needs and preferences by avoiding those you don't like, fitting them into your personal schedule, and so forth. Do these things and you are eating just like the world's fittest people.

Of course, I am not recommending that you actually limit your future eating to these seventeen recipes. But the more you draw from them, the easier it may be for you to find your initial footing on the Endurance Diet. In addition to supplying you with specific meals that are consistent with Endurance Diet standards, the recipes can serve as a template for other meal choices. From this point forward, you will want to eat meals like these, if not these meals specifically.

All of the recipes were created by my longtime collaborator Georgie Fear in response to my request for a selection of dishes that broadly represent what elite endurance athletes eat in various parts of the world. Most of them contain one or more of the endurance superfoods identified in Chapter 10; these appear in **boldface**. I think you will be as impressed with the things she came up with as I was. For more recipes like them, check out our *Racing Weight Cookbook*.

Note that, although I've emphasized that counting calories and monitoring nutrients is generally unimportant in the Endurance Diet, basic nutrition facts for all recipes are included. This information may help you with such things as keeping your diet carb-centered and maintaining a higher protein intake during weight-loss focus phases.

Endurance Diet Recipes

1. Custard Oats with Fruit and Pecans
2. Zesty Green Smoothie
3. Bagel Breakfast Sandwich
4. Blini with Cherry-Blueberry-Maple Topping
5. Broiled Vegetable Panini with Edamame Hummus
6. Kickin' Turkey Cheeseburgers
7. Fish Tacos
8. Lohikeitto (Salmon Soup)
9. Chicken Stir-Fry with Honey-Ginger Sauce
10. Beef and Soba Noodle Bowl with Almond Butter–Chile Sauce
11. Whole Wheat Spaghetti and Bison Meatballs
12. Slow Cooker Cuban Black Beans and Rice
13. Moroccan Stew
14. Ugali with Sukuma Wiki
15. Southwest Chili with One-Bowl Cornbread
16. Ratatouille
17. Shepherd's Pie

Custard Oats with Fruit and Pecans
(Scotland)

Full of complex carbohydrates and fiber, oatmeal is a great nutritional kick-starter for the day, especially when it includes nuts, seeds, and fruit. This version gets an added protein punch from egg whites, which will help you stay full for longer and give the dish an appealing custardy texture.

1/2 cup water
1/2 cup unsweetened almond milk (any variety or fat level will work, including other nondairy milks)

Pinch of salt

2 teaspoons brown sugar

1 **banana**, sliced, divided

1/2 cup oatmeal (old-fashioned oats)

1/3 cup **egg whites** (pasteurized from a carton is easiest, or use the whites of 2 eggs)

1 tablespoon chopped pecans

1/4 cup blueberries

1. Combine water, milk, salt, brown sugar, and half of the sliced banana in a saucepan and bring to a boil over medium heat.
2. Add oatmeal and stir. Cook for 5 minutes or until oatmeal is thickened, stirring occasionally.
3. Add the egg whites and immediately begin stirring for one full minute.
4. Turn off heat, transfer to a bowl, and top with remaining banana slices, pecans, and blueberries.

Serves 1

Nutrition Facts: 411 calories, 9 g total fat, 68 g total carb, 9 g fiber, 17 g protein

Zesty Green Smoothie
(North America)

Any protein powder you have on hand will work in this smoothie, a powerhouse blend of polyphenol-rich green tea, vitamin-packed leafy greens, nitrate-rich celery, and fresh fruit. You'll benefit as well from a hefty dose of vitamin C and potassium from the kiwi and banana, essentials for replacing minerals lost in sweat and healing soft-tissue wear and tear. For best results, use a high-speed blender for this recipe.

1 stick celery

1 small piece peeled fresh ginger (about half the size of a little finger)

1 cup cold water or chilled **green tea**

1 handful dark leafy greens (**spinach**, kale, sprouts)

1/4 avocado

1 scoop Optimum Nutrition Vanilla Whey Protein Powder

1 kiwi

1 **banana**

Combine all ingredients in a blender pitcher and blend until smooth.

Serves 1

Nutrition Facts: 359 calories, 8 g total fat, 49 g total carb, 10 g fiber, 29 g protein

Bagel Breakfast Sandwich
(North America)

A typical breakfast sandwich is reliable as a source of grains, eggs, and fat from either bacon or cheese. But it's likely to be missing whole grains and rarely if ever does it contain vegetables. We've got those nutritional bases covered, however, with this tasty and colorful utensil-free breakfast delight.

1 whole-grain bagel

Olive oil or canola oil cooking spray

1 **egg**

Salt and pepper to taste

1 handful baby **spinach**

1 ounce nitrate-free deli ham

1 ounce roasted red pepper (from a jar)

1 slice cheddar or pepper jack cheese

1. Preheat oven or toaster oven to 400 degrees and lightly oil a baking sheet (or use a nonstick mat). Slice bagel in half and place cut side up on the baking sheet. Place in oven for 5 minutes or until lightly toasted.

2. Lightly coat a skillet with cooking spray, and place over medium heat. Crack egg into the center of the pan, season to taste with salt and pepper and cook uncovered for 1 minute. This will begin to cook the white part. The yolk will not set until it's covered and steamed. Then, add the spinach around the outside of the pan (or wherever there is room) and cover the pan so the egg steams and the spinach wilts. Check the yolk every minute or two and remove the egg and spinach from the pan when it reaches your desired degree of doneness.

3. Place the red pepper and ham on one bagel half, and the cheese on the other half, and return to oven for 2–3 minutes to melt cheese and heat up ham and red pepper. One half may need a minute or two longer than the other.

4. Assemble sandwich by placing the fried egg and wilted spinach on the pepper and ham side, and topping it with the cheesy bagel half.

Serves 1

Nutrition Facts: 464 calories, 14 g total fat, 62 g total carb, 4 g fiber, 25 g protein

Blini with Cherry-Blueberry-Maple Topping
(Russia)

Buckwheat flour gives these small pancakes a rich amber color and a pleasing nutty flavor. To keep the added sugars moderate, we use flavonoid-packed fruit for the topping, with just enough genuine maple syrup (which does not subtract points from your Diet Quality Score when used in moderation) to keep it from being too tart. The flavor of genuine maple syrup is more intense than that of the imitations sold at supermarkets, which allows you to use less.

1/2 cup fresh or frozen pitted **cherries**
1/2 cup fresh or frozen blueberries
1 tablespoon real maple syrup
1/3 cup buckwheat flour
1/3 cup whole wheat flour
1 teaspoon baking powder
1/4 teaspoon salt
1/2 teaspoon sugar
1 **egg**
2/3 cup whole milk (nondairy milks will work as well)
1 teaspoon canola oil or melted butter
Plain **yogurt** or sour cream, optional, for serving.

1. In a small saucepan, combine cherries, blueberries, and maple syrup. Place over low heat to simmer gently while you make the blini.
2. Combine flours, baking powder, salt, and sugar in a large bowl and whisk to blend. The batter should be fairly thin and lump-free.
3. Add egg, milk, and oil, and whisk or stir to blend.
4. Heat a nonstick skillet over medium heat for 1 minute. Pour batter into 2- to 3-inch circles, leaving room between so they don't run into each other.
5. When bubbles appear across the surface of the pancakes, flip them over and cook 1–2 minutes on the other side or until they easily remove from pan.
6. Repeat to use up all the batter.
7. Serve blini with berry topping and plain yogurt or sour cream, if desired.

Makes 15–20 blini (2 to 3 inches across).

Serves 2 as a meal

Nutrition Facts: 380 calories, 9 g total fat, 64 g total carb, 9 g fiber, 15 g protein

Broiled Vegetable Panini with Edamame Hummus
(Italy/Greece)

Hummus is traditionally made from chickpeas, but this version is unique in its use of green soybeans, also known as edamame, for a protein boost and a lovely green hue. Use leftover hummus for dipping raw veggies.

1 large red pepper, cut into three to four pieces
1 Japanese eggplant (long, thin kind) cut into 1/4-inch slices diagonally
1 medium zucchini, cut into 1/4-inch slices diagonally
Olive oil or canola oil cooking spray
Sea salt
Black pepper
4 slices whole-grain bread
2 slices Havarti cheese
3 tablespoons edamame hummus (recipe below) or store-bought hummus

1. Preheat broiler and place a rack in the oven 3–4 inches from heating element. Line a baking sheet with tin foil and coat it with cooking spray (alternatively, use a nonstick baking mat).
2. Arrange red pepper, eggplant, and zucchini slices on the lined baking sheet. Mist the vegetables lightly with cooking spray and season with sea salt and black pepper.
3. Broil vegetables for 5 minutes, then remove from oven and flip pieces with a pancake turner. Broil 5 minutes more, then remove from oven and turn off broiler. If the skin on the peppers is charred and black, remove it after they have cooled enough to touch without burning your fingers.

4. Toast the bread and spread two slices each with 1 1/2 tablespoons hummus. These are the base of each sandwich.

5. Place a slice of cheese on top of the hummus, then layer on approximately half the broiled vegetables onto each sandwich, topping with remaining slice of toasted bread.

6. If desired, press sandwiches in panini press or indoor (George Foreman–style) grill.

Serves 2

Nutrition Facts: 378 calories, 14 g total fat, 56 g total carb, 13 g fiber, 18 g protein

Edamame Hummus

1 cup shelled edamame
2 tablespoons fresh lemon juice
2 tablespoons water
2 tablespoons extra-virgin **olive oil**
1/4 teaspoon salt
1/4 teaspoon garlic powder
1/8 teaspoon black pepper

Combine all ingredients in a food processor and process until smooth. Store in refrigerator up to one week.

Makes 3/4 cup hummus (8 servings, 1 1/2 tablespoons each).
Nutrition Facts: 58 calories, 4 g total fat, 3 g total carb, 2 g fiber, 2 g protein

Kickin' Turkey Cheeseburgers
(North America)

We flavored these turkey burgers with a fun combination of Worcestershire sauce, mustard, and green onion, plus hot sauce for a bit of kick.

If you like a little spice on your palate, you'll love this creative take on an American classic. Almost any cheese is a perfect accompaniment; bold cheddar and creamy Monterey Jack are just two of our favorites.

- 1 pound ground turkey
- 1/2 cup finely diced green onion, green and white parts (about five)
- 1/2 teaspoon salt
- 1/4 teaspoon black pepper
- 2 teaspoons Worcestershire sauce
- 2 teaspoons hot sauce or Sriracha
- 2 teaspoons prepared mustard (Dijon or yellow)
- 1 **egg**
- 3 slices cheddar or Monterey Jack cheese

Mix all ingredients except cheese in a medium bowl and form into three burgers. Grill or pan fry for 6–7 minutes per side, or until internal temperature reaches 165 degrees F. Top with cheese.

Serves 3

Nutrition Facts: 278 calories, 15 g total fat, 3 g total carb, 1 g fiber, 32 g protein

Fish Tacos
(Mexico)

Many fish tacos you get at restaurants are deep fried, but not this version. Simple seasonings of cumin and cayenne give the fish a savory heat, and the lime juice and coleslaw mix (shredded cabbage and carrots) finish the dish with freshness and just a little crunch. If you like, you can substitute jicama for the coleslaw mix.

- 1 pound white fish such as bass or cod
- 1/2 teaspoon cumin
- 1/4–1/2 teaspoon cayenne pepper (depending on your spice preference)

1/4 teaspoon salt
1/4 teaspoon black pepper
1 tablespoon lime juice
6 small whole wheat tortillas
1 cup coleslaw mix, undressed
1/2 cup fresh cilantro leaves
Salsa

1. Place fish in a nonstick skillet and sprinkle evenly with cumin, cayenne, salt, and pepper. Cover and cook over medium heat for 6 minutes or until fish is opaque and flakes easily. Turn off heat. Flake fish into chunks with a spatula or wooden spoon and sprinkle with lime juice.
2. Divide fish among tortillas and top with coleslaw mix and cilantro. Serve with salsa.

Serves 2

Nutrition Facts: 427 calories, 9 g total fat, 46 g total carb, 8 g fiber, 40 g protein

Lohikeitto (Salmon Soup)
(Finland)

Finnish food is simple, hearty, and warming, and this soup stays true to those themes. Instead of using all fresh salmon, which would have been the conventional choice, we've included a small amount of smoked salmon to give another layer of flavor to the dish.

1 leek, sliced
1 onion, chopped (yellow or white)
1/2 tablespoon extra-virgin **olive oil**
1 pound white nugget **potatoes** (8 small) cut into 1-inch pieces
    (peel, if desired, but I don't)

1 carrot, diced

2 cups vegetable or fish broth, plus 2 cups water

12 ounces wild **salmon**, skinned and cut into 1- to 2-inch cubes

4 ounces smoked **salmon**, cut into 1 inch pieces

1 cup whole milk or half and half

1 cup chopped fresh dill (about 1 ounce)

salt (I used 1/2 teaspoon)

black pepper (1/2 teaspoon)

4 slices rye bread, optional, for serving

1. In a medium pot, cook onion and leek in olive oil over medium heat until softened, about 8 minutes.
2. Add potatoes, carrot, broth, and water and cover. Turn heat to high to bring to a boil, then reduce to medium for 5 minutes or until potatoes are tender.
3. Turn heat to low. Add both types of salmon and simmer for 5 minutes. From this point only stir very gently to avoid breaking up salmon.
4. Add milk, dill, and salt and pepper to taste. Remove from heat and serve with toasted rye bread.

Serves 4

Nutrition Facts: 291 calories, 7 g total fat, 32 g total carb, 4 g fiber, 29 g protein (served without bread, made with whole milk).

334 calories, 12 g fat, 31 g carb, 29 g protein (made with half and half)

Chicken Stir-Fry with Honey-Ginger Sauce
(China)

Asian food is known for blending sweet, spicy, salty, and savory flavors, but in the West it is also often associated with deep-fried items tossed in a large amount of sugary sauce. Our version of the chicken stir-fry contains plenty of flavor with just enough honey to give it a sweet note. You can use this recipe with other proteins such as tofu, beef, shrimp, or pork.

4 teaspoons soy sauce
4 teaspoons white vinegar
2 teaspoons honey
1/2 teaspoon hot red pepper flakes
1 teaspoon cornstarch
1 teaspoon canola, sesame, or coconut oil
3/4 pound boneless skinless chicken breast, cut into bite-sized
    pieces
salt and pepper
1/2 cup water
2 small or 1 large broccoli crown, cut into florets
1 inch piece of fresh ginger, peeled and minced
3 **garlic** cloves, minced
6 shiitake mushrooms, sliced
1 yellow bell pepper, sliced
2 cups cooked **brown rice**

1. In a small bowl, stir together soy sauce, vinegar, honey, red pepper flakes, and cornstarch. Set aside.
2. Heat a large skillet or wok over medium heat for one minute and add oil. Skillet is ready when drops of water sizzle on it.
3. Add chicken to hot pan and season lightly with salt and pepper. Cook for 4–5 minutes, tossing every minute or so, over medium-high heat until outside of chicken is golden and pieces are cooked through. Transfer to a platter and return skillet to heat.
4. Place broccoli and 1/2 cup of water into skillet and cover. Cook 3 minutes, then remove lid and add ginger, garlic, mushrooms, and yellow pepper.

5. Cook and stir vegetables until water has evaporated, about 1–2 minutes, then add sauce to skillet. Allow sauce to boil for 1 minute and thicken, then return cooked chicken to skillet and gently mix everything together to coat with sauce.
6. Serve stir-fry atop cooked rice.

Serves 2

Nutrition Facts: 548 calories, 9 g total fat, 75 g total carb, 12 g fiber, 49 g protein (including rice)

Beef and Soba Noodle Bowl with Almond Butter–Chile Sauce
(Japan)

The star of this recipe is the sauce, which you may find yourself making again and again to put on other dishes. It's sweet, spicy, and salty, and the almond butter (endurance superfood!) gives it a flavor you won't find in more traditional noodle dishes.

4 ounces soba noodles
3 cloves **garlic**, minced
1 inch piece of fresh ginger, peeled and minced
8 ounces extra-lean ground beef
2 1/2 tablespoons soy sauce
1 1/2 tablespoons **almond butter**
2 tablespoons Sriracha hot sauce (reduce to one if you are sensitive to spice)
1 teaspoon cornstarch
1 tablespoon honey
1/3 cup water
7 ounces sugar snap peas or snow peas
5 ounces matchstick cut carrots (half a 10 ounce bag)
3 green onions, sliced (white and green parts)
hot pepper flakes, optional, for garnish

1. Bring 4 cups of water to a boil. Cook soba noodles according to package directions, drain, and set aside.

2. Combine garlic, ginger, and beef in a large nonstick pan and cook over medium heat, breaking up beef with a wooden or silicone spatula, until no pink color remains, about 8–10 minutes. Do *not* reduce or remove from heat before moving to the next step.

3. In a small bowl, combine soy sauce, almond butter, Sriracha, cornstarch, and honey. Stir to blend and pour into beef mixture. Add 1/3 cup water and continue to cook over medium heat until sauce bubbles for about 1 minute and thickens.

4. Add snap peas, carrots, and green onions to pan with beef, and stir gently to mix. Cook, stirring occasionally, until carrots and snap peas are tender, about 4 minutes. Add cooked soba and gently mix.

5. Divide between two bowls and garnish with hot red pepper flakes or a squiggle of Sriracha.

Serves 2

Nutrition Facts: 574 calories, 13 g total fat, 74 g total carb, 9 g fiber, 41 g protein

Whole Wheat Spaghetti and Bison Meatballs
(Italy)

More than one of our athletes have set personal records after having this satisfying dish for dinner the night before. We can't promise it will do the same for you, but so far no one has ever been slowed down by it! Classic spaghetti and meatballs gets a flavor and nutrition upgrade in this version from the substitution of lean bison meat for beef, and the addition of a hearty serving of vegetables to the sauce. Chase this with a good night's sleep and you'll be ready to rock in the morning.

1 pound lean ground bison
1 **egg**

1/2 cup finely minced onion (yellow or white)

2 cloves **garlic**, minced

1/2 teaspoon Italian seasoning

1 teaspoon salt

1/2 teaspoon black pepper

1/4 teaspoon red pepper flakes, optional

1 pound whole wheat spaghetti

1 large orange or yellow bell pepper, chopped

1 medium zucchini, chopped

1 cup sliced mushrooms

3 cups prepared **tomato** sauce

1. Combine bison, egg, onion, garlic, Italian seasoning, salt, black pepper, and red pepper flakes in a large bowl and mix well by hand.
2. Roll into balls, each one slightly bigger than a golf ball. It should yield about twelve meatballs. Place formed meatballs in a large skillet in a single layer.
3. When all the meatballs are formed, place the skillet over medium heat. Cover to minimize splattering, and cook for 10 minutes, gently turning every few minutes to brown the meatballs on all sides.
4. With lid slightly ajar, drain liquid from the pan. Add bell pepper, zucchini, mushrooms, and tomato sauce. Simmer for 15 minutes.
5. While sauce and meatballs cook, boil pasta according to package direction.
6. Serve meatballs and sauce over cooked and drained spaghetti.

Serves 4

Nutrition Facts: 575 calories, 17 g total fat, 68 g total carb, 11 g fiber, 39 g protein

Slow Cooker Cuban Black Beans and Rice
(Cuba)

This Cuban classic offers an easy, delicious way to incorporate an endurance superfood into your meals. This comfort food recipe will give you several servings of warm, carbohydrate-rich yumminess. A plate of black beans and rice is a perfect recovery meal to come home to after a long workout when you don't want to spend time laboring in the kitchen, or as a quick warmer-upper after a cold day outside. We added a jalapeño, which is not an ingredient in the authentic Cuban dish, but you can omit it if you prefer.

Note: the recipe calls for dry beans; if you want to use canned, use four 15-ounce cans of no-salt-added beans, rinsed and drained. You'll also want to reduce the water by one cup.

16 ounces dry **black beans**
1 large onion, chopped
1 large bell pepper, chopped (any color)
6 **garlic** cloves, minced
1 jalapeño pepper, chopped (seeds removed)
1 (28 ounce) can diced **tomatoes**, undrained
3 1/2 cups water
2 tablespoons **olive oil**
2 tablespoons red wine vinegar
1/2 teaspoon ground cumin
1/2 teaspoon dried oregano
2 dried bay leaves
1 teaspoon salt
3 cups **brown rice**

1. Rinse black beans and drain. Place in slow cooker with all other ingredients except the rice. Stir and cover.
2. Cook on high heat setting for 6–8 hours or until beans are tender and most liquid is absorbed. Remove bay leaves.

3. Cook rice according to package directions. Serve black beans atop rice.

Serves 9

Nutrition Facts: (1 cup beans with 1 cup rice): 417 calories, 5 g total fat, 79 g carb, 20 g dietary fiber, 15 g protein

Moroccan Stew
(Morocco)

Virtually all the work required to make this stew consists of chopping up the ingredients; after that you just toss everything in a pot and let it simmer. Enjoy this stew on its own, or serve with whole wheat couscous for extra carbs.

1 cup chopped onions (1 medium)
1 cup diced celery (2 ribs)
1 cup chopped green bell pepper (1 medium)
2 cup chopped carrots (4-5 large)
2 cloves of **garlic**, minced
1 inch piece ginger root, peeled and minced
1 medium **sweet potato**, chopped
3 cups vegetable or chicken broth
2 teaspoons each ground cumin, curry powder, and ground coriander
1/4 teaspoon cayenne pepper (more if desired)
1 can (19 ounces/540 milliliters) diced **tomatoes**, drained
1 can (19 ounces/540 milliliters) chickpeas, drained and rinsed
4 cups (packed) chopped kale (yield from one bunch, stems removed)
1/4 cup all-natural **peanut butter**
1/4 cup light or dark raisins, optional
Optional couscous, for serving

Heat a large pot over medium-high heat. Add everything except kale, peanut butter, and raisins. Bring to a boil and reduce heat to low. Simmer for 10 minutes or until potatoes are tender. Stir in kale, peanut butter, and raisins. Simmer for 5 minutes more. Taste and add additional cayenne to reach desired level of spice. Serve hot.

Serves 4

Nutrition Facts: 406 calories, 10 g total fat, 68 g total carb, 17 g fiber, 17 g protein (without couscous)

Ugali with Sukuma Wiki
(Kenya)

Traditionally, this meal, like most traditional Kenyan food, is eaten with the hands: you tear off a small piece of ugali and form it into a ball with a depression in it. You then use the ugali to scoop up the greens (sukuma wiki) or whatever stew or meat is served alongside it. These greens can also be enjoyed with chapati, or flatbreads. Feel free to add any leftover meat to the greens in step two to provide additional protein, or add a side of canned beans for a vegan protein.

Ugali
  1 cup **corn** flour (white or yellow)
  2 cups water
  pinch salt

Sukuma Wiki
  2 teaspoons **olive oil**
  1 white onion
  1/2 teaspoon cumin
  1/2 teaspoon coriander
  1/8 teaspoon cayenne pepper
  2 plum **tomatoes**, chopped

1 pound kale or collard greens (2 bunches), stems removed and
shredded or chopped

1 cup water

1/4 teaspoon salt (or to taste)

1/8 teaspoon black pepper (or to taste)

1 lemon

1. Sauté onion in olive oil over medium heat until soft, for 8 minutes. Add cumin, coriander, cayenne, and tomatoes and stir.

2. One handful at a time, add shredded collards or kale, stirring to coat with other ingredients. Add water and cover. Cook 30 minutes or until greens reach your desired tenderness.

3. While greens are cooking, bring 2 cups of water and a pinch of salt to a boil in a saucepan. Turn heat to low, and slowly add corn flour, stirring continuously to break up lumps. Continue to cook and stir for 3 to 4 minutes or until mixture is a stiff porridge. Turn off heat and scoop into a serving bowl.

4. When greens are cooked, season with salt and pepper to taste. Serve sukuma wiki alongside ugali, with a lemon wedge to squeeze some fresh lemon juice on each portion of greens.

Serves 4

Nutrition Facts: 159 calories, 4 g total fat, 30 g total carb, 5 g fiber, 4 g protein

Southwest Chili with One-Bowl Cornbread
(North America)

If you prefer a traditional style of chili, you are sure to enjoy this recipe, which hews close to the classic seasoning profile for the beloved Southwest American dish, with a deeper flavor note from the unsweetened cocoa. Feel free to toss in corn kernels or swap black beans for kidney beans as you prefer.

1 pound extra-lean ground beef or bison

1 1/2 cups chopped bell peppers (red, green, yellow)

1/2 large yellow onion, chopped

3 cloves **garlic**

1 tablespoon ground cumin

1 tablespoon unsweetened cocoa powder

2 1/2 tablespoons chili powder

1/2 teaspoon cayenne pepper, or more to taste

2 cans (14 ounces) diced **tomatoes**

19-ounce can kidney beans, drained and rinsed

Salt to taste

Fresh cilantro for topping

1. In a saucepan with lid, cook ground beef or bison over medium heat while breaking up with a wooden spoon. Cook until no pink remains, about 8-10 minutes. Drain fat, if any, and return meat crumbles to pot.

2. Add bell peppers, onion, garlic, cumin, cocoa, chili powder, cayenne pepper, diced tomatoes (with their liquid), and beans to pot. Stir to blend.

3. Cover and when mixture begins to bubble, reduce heat to low. Simmer for 30–45 minutes. Add salt to taste.

4. Serve sprinkled with fresh cilantro.

Serves 4

Nutrition Facts: 335 calories, 5 g total fat, 36 g total carb, 11 g fiber, 38 g protein

One-Bowl Cornbread

1 1/4 cups **cornmeal**

1 cup whole wheat flour

1 tablespoon baking powder

1/2 teaspoon baking soda

1/3 cup sugar

1/2 teaspoon salt

1 **egg**

2 tablespoons melted butter or coconut oil

1 cup skim milk or unsweetened almond milk

2 tablespoons plain or vanilla Greek **yogurt**

1. Preheat oven to 400 degrees. Oil the inside of a 9- or 10-inch cast iron skillet. (Use a cake pan if you don't have a cast iron skillet.)
2. In a large mixing bowl, combine cornmeal, flour, baking powder, baking soda, sugar, and salt and stir to mix.
3. Add egg, butter or oil, milk, and yogurt and stir just until uniformly mixed. Pour batter into prepared skillet and bake 15 minutes or until knife inserted in the center comes out clean.

Serves 8

Nutrition Facts: 219 calories, 6 g total fat, 35 g total carb, 3 g fiber, 5 g protein

Ratatouille
(France)

This classic French recipe will happily simmer on your stovetop or in your slow cooker while you're out biking in the Alps in preparation for the Tour (or swimming laps at the local Y, or whatever). Don't forget the crusty bread; it's vital to the full experience. Feta isn't exactly traditional, but it is a nice twist if you have it on hand.

1 tablespoon extra-virgin **olive oil**

1 sweet onion, chopped

5 **garlic** cloves, chopped

1 red pepper, cut into 1-inch pieces

1 yellow pepper, cut into 1-inch pieces

1 pound of zucchini, cut into 1-inch pieces

1 medium eggplant (1 pound) cut into 1-inch pieces

1 1/2 pounds **tomatoes**, cut into 1-inch pieces (5–6 tomatoes)

1/2 teaspoon each: salt, red pepper flakes, dried thyme

4 tablespoons no-salt-added **tomato** paste

1/2 cup fresh basil leaves, shredded (1/4 cup after shredding)

2 ounces grated parmesan or crumbled feta

Crusty whole-grain bread

1. Combine all ingredients except basil, cheese, and bread in a large soup pot or Dutch oven. Cover and bring to a boil over high heat, then reduce heat to low and simmer for 45–60 minutes or until vegetables are soft.
2. Alternatively, this dish can be cooked in a slow cooker for 6–8 hours on low.
3. Top each serving with a pinch of shredded basil and 1/2 ounce grated parmesan or crumbled feta. Serve with crusty whole-grain bread.

Serves 6

Nutrition Facts (without bread): 118 calories, 5 g total fat, 16 g total carb, 5 g fiber, 5 g protein

Nutrition Facts (with bread): 258 calories, 6 g total fat, 44 g total carb, 8 g fiber, 11 g protein

Shepherd's Pie
(Great Britain)

Seasoned lamb and vegetables under a blanket of mashed potatoes is classic British home cooking, but traditional shepherd's pies contain more fat and less carbohydrate than is ideal for endurance athletes in training. We've tweaked the macronutrient ratio of our version without sacrificing taste with modifications such as using Greek yogurt in place of some of the butter and whole milk.

Filling:
 1 pound ground lamb
 2 celery ribs, chopped
 1 yellow onion, chopped
 2 carrots, chopped
 2 cloves **garlic**, minced
 2 tablespoons Worcestershire sauce
 1/4 cup **tomato** sauce
 1/2 teaspoon black pepper
 1/4 teaspoon salt
 1/2 teaspoon dried thyme
 1 cup frozen green peas

Mashed potato topping:
 2 pounds russet **potatoes**
 1/3 cup milk
 1/3 cup Greek **yogurt**
 1 tablespoon butter
 salt and pepper to taste

1. Cut potatoes into 2-inch chunks and place in a pot. Cover with water and bring to a boil. Cook until tender and easily pierced with a fork, about 20–25 minutes, while you prepare the filling.
2. Preheat oven to 400 degrees F. Place an oven-proof 10-inch skillet (cast iron is our preference) over medium heat and add the lamb, celery, onion, carrot, and garlic.
3. Cook and break up meat until lamb is completely browned, about 8–10 minutes. Place a lid over the pan and drain liquid. (Alternatively, push vegetables and meat to one side and spoon out grease.)

4. Add Worcestershire sauce, tomato sauce, pepper, salt, thyme, and peas to pan and stir to blend. Smooth evenly in skillet and turn off heat.

5. Drain the potatoes and mash with milk, yogurt, and butter, and add salt and pepper to taste. Spread the mashed potatoes over lamb–vegetable mixture and bake for 30 minutes.

Serves 4

Nutrition Facts: 477 calories, 17 g total fat, 55 g total carb, 8 g fiber, 33 g protein

12   Diet–Exercise Synergy

YOU ARE *NOT* WHAT YOU EAT. YOU ARE *WHAT YOUR BODY DOES WITH* WHAT you eat. And what your body does with what you eat is strongly influenced by what you do with your body. Any given diet will generate very different outcomes in a person who does not exercise than it will in a person who does. The same diet will even generate different outcomes in two people who exercise but in different ways.

The term *diet–exercise synergy* refers to the idea that diet mediates the effects of exercise and vice versa. Our main interest in this book has been the diet side of this equation. My goal in the preceding chapters was to describe the diet habits that maximize the fitness-boosting effects of endurance exercise and to supply all of the guidance you need to practice this way of eating.

Now imagine yourself practicing the Endurance Diet flawlessly for six months and not doing a single workout during this period of time. How fit would you be at the end of it? Not very! Nor would you have a very high level of endurance fitness if you practiced the Endurance Diet flawlessly for six months and did only yoga or bodybuilding workouts.

The point of these thought experiments is to highlight the fact that practicing the Endurance Diet is not sufficient in itself to maximize endurance fitness. You need to exercise as conscientiously as you eat to become as fit as you can be. In this sense, the Endurance Diet is not complete without proper endurance training. Or, put another way, proper training is a part of the Endurance Diet. For this reason, I think it's appropriate to conclude this book with some guidance on training.

Like the five eating habits that collectively optimize endurance fitness, the training methods that do the same were not deduced by scientists but instead evolved through a long-term process of trial and error carried out by elite athletes and coaches around the world. The difference is that there is more sport-specific particularity in the training methods of elite endurance athletes than there is in their diets. For example, elite swimmers typically swim twice a day and do a lot of technique work, whereas elite cyclists ride their bikes just once a day and spend little time working on technique. Yet the diets of elite swimmers and cyclists are virtually indistinguishable.

Nevertheless, the various endurance sport disciplines are similar enough in their physical demands that a shared set of core training methods has proved to be optimal in all of them. In the next section, I will describe eight such methods. Like the Endurance Diet, these optimal training methods are practiced far less often by recreational endurance athletes and exercisers than they are by the professionals. Incorporating any of these methods that you do not currently practice into your training will increase your fitness level and ensure that no portion of your optimal eating habits is wasted.

It should be noted that some methods are more relevant to athletes whose primary goal is peak performance in competitive events than they are to exercisers who work out for other reasons. Throughout this book I have addressed athletes and exercisers collectively because both groups seek endurance fitness and the same diet that is most effective for performance maximizes its health benefits also. But where training is concerned, athletes and exercisers are different.

The key difference is that athletes aim to "peak" for races—that is, to attain the very highest possible level of fitness on just a handful of isolated days each year. This orientation demands a variable approach to training in which athletes push themselves very hard at some times, prioritize rest at other times, and carefully sequence their workouts in such a way that they are always moving toward their next fitness target. Exercisers, on the other hand, are more interested in consistency. Most noncompetitive cardio buffs train progressively to the point where they are satisfied with their results and then try to hold steady. For this reason, training methods such as periodization (the exercise counterpart to nutritional periodization, discussed in Chapter 9) that are essential for athletes are not essential for exercisers.

It's important not to confuse this distinction of types with the spectrum of "seriousness." There are casual athletes who take a minimalist approach to training and don't mind finishing races at the back of the pack and there are very serious noncompetitive exercisers who train harder than most athletes and look like they could win races if they ever chose to enter any.

It bears mentioning as well that the athlete/exerciser distinction is fungible. An athlete and an exerciser may be the same person at different times. Most athletes start off as exercisers (indeed, I enjoy nothing more than turning exercisers into athletes) and athletes often take breaks from competition for a period of time without giving up exercise.

In the following descriptions of the eight training methods that are essential for maximum endurance fitness, I will focus mainly on the interests of athletes but will conclude each section with a few words about the method's relevance to noncompetitive exercisers. If you're an exerciser who gets the urge to become an athlete or an athlete who needs a break from competition, simply switch from one set of guidelines to the other.

Eight Essential Training Methods for Maximum Endurance Fitness

Just as eating individually is a key part of the optimal diet for endurance fitness, so too is training individually a key part of the optimal exercise program for endurance fitness. For example, some athletes need more time to recover from high-intensity intervals than others do and therefore must plan out their weekly workout schedule accordingly. Experience will reveal what works best for you.

Such individual differences occur at the level of details, however. There is a core foundation of best practices in endurance training that are the same for all athletes. Think of these eight practices as the rules that you cannot get away with breaking if you want to get the greatest possible benefit from the time and energy you invest in working out.

The 80/20 Rule

The foundation of optimal training for endurance fitness is an appropriate intensity balance. Intensity is simply how hard you are exercising at a given moment relative to your personal limit. Research conducted mostly within the past decade has demonstrated that endurance athletes of all experience and ability levels gain the most fitness when they spend approximately 80 percent of their total training time at low intensity and the remaining 20 percent at moderate to high intensity.

Nearly all elite endurance athletes obey the 80/20 Rule of intensity balance, but very few recreational athletes do. A 1993 study by researchers at Arizona State University found that competitive recreational runners did only 46 percent of their training at low intensity and another 46 percent at moderate intensity. And, in 2012, Stuart Galloway and colleagues at the University of Stirling in Scotland reported that a group of recreational triathletes training for an Ironman event did less than 70 percent of their training at low intensity.

Other research has shown that this training error is not only common but also costly. In controlled studies in which some athletes follow the 80/20 Rule and others don't, the former always improve more. For example, in a 2014 experiment led by Jonathan Esteve-Lanao, fifteen club-level Spanish runners followed the 80/20 Rule while another fifteen maintained a 50/50 split (as most recreational runners do). After ten weeks, the runners in the 50/50 group had lowered their 10K time by an average of 3.5 percent, which is not bad. But the runners who followed the 80/20 Rule most faithfully improved by *double* that amount.

Escaping the "moderate-intensity rut" that most recreational endurance athletes are stuck in and falling in line with the 80/20 Rule is a three-step process.

Step 1: Learn to distinguish among low, moderate, and high intensities. Physiologically, the borderline between low and moderate intensity falls at 96 percent of the highest heart rate you could sustain for one hour. The borderline between moderate and high intensity falls at 102 percent of this heart rate.

To determine your personal low-intensity (LI), moderate-intensity (MI), and high-intensity (HI) training zones, warm up and then settle into the highest speed or power output you believe you could sustain for one hour. Wait for your heart rate to plateau and then note it. Subtract 4 percent from this number to determine your low-intensity ceiling. Add 2 percent to the same number to determine your moderate-intensity ceiling.

Step 2: Plan your training so that roughly 80 percent of your total weekly training time is spent at low intensity. This is a simple game of math. For example, if you exercise five hours per week, that's 300 minutes. Eighty percent of 300 is 240, or four hours. Here's how a five-hour training week with one hour of moderate- and high-intensity training might look:

Monday	Tuesday	Wednesday	Thursday	Friday	Saturday	Sunday
	15:00 LI 30:00 MI 15:00 LI	45:00 LI	45:00 LI	10:00 LI 6 x (5:00 HI/2:30 LI) 5:00 LI	30:00 LI	90:00 LI

Step 3: Execution. It's one thing to plan the perfect 80/20 week, another to actually do it. If you're like many endurance athletes and exercisers, you already *intend* to do most of your training at low intensity, but when you get out on the road or the water, you do something else—without even realizing it. Fixing this problem requires what Stephen Seiler, the aforementioned discoverer of the 80/20 Rule, calls "intensity discipline." Training with a heart rate monitor is helpful in this regard. Once you've established the heart rates that correspond to low, moderate, and high intensity for you, it's easy to stay in the right zone by keeping an eye on your monitor.

Understand that there is no magic in round numbers. It is not necessary to do *exactly* 80 percent of your training at low intensity. In fact, there is no need to follow the 80/20 Rule at all except when you are aiming toward maximum fitness—for example in the 12 or 16 weeks before a race. During "base" training, when you are really preparing just to prepare for maximum fitness, it may be best to spend even less than 20 percent of your total training time at moderate to high intensity.

Note that the 80/20 Rule says nothing about the best way to balance moderate- and high-intensity training. Stephen Seiler favors a "polarized" approach, in which most of the 80 percent of training that is not done at low intensity is done at high intensity. My own view is that, for competitive athletes, the optimal balance depends on the distance of the races being preparing for. The longer they are, the more the balance should tilt from high intensity to moderate intensity.

The 80/20 Rule is relevant to exercisers as well as athletes. Even if you don't compete, you will get the biggest fitness bang for your workout buck if you spend four minutes out of every five at low intensity. The exception is when you care more about fat loss than any other outcome of exercising, such as during a weight-loss focus phase. In this case, a high-intensity interval-based program in which as much as half of total training time is spent at high intensity and the overall volume of training is relatively low is likely to be most effective.

Progressive Overload

The principle of progressive overload is based on the idea that fitness improves most reliably when the body is consistently (though not uninterruptedly) exposed to slightly greater exercise challenges than it is accustomed to. Applying this principle to the training process generally entails making each week of training a little harder than the one before—either by increasing the overall amount of exercise or by holding the total amount of exercise steady and increasing the fraction of total workout time that is spent at higher intensities—except in recovery weeks, which I will discuss below.

The alternatives to progressive overload are (1) repeating the same training every week, (2) increasing the training load drastically from week to week, and (3) decreasing the training load from week to week. Each alternative is inferior to progressive overload in its own way.

Repeating the same training from week to week: This will keep you at your current fitness level but won't make you any fitter, even if you work out a lot. Fitness is an adaptation to stress, after all, and stress comes from challenging the body more than it is accustomed to. A swimmer who has not swum more than nine thousand yards in a week recently will get a fitness-boosting stimulus from swimming ten thousand yards next week, but a swimmer who swims ten thousand yards per week routinely will not.

Increasing the training load drastically from week to week: This will overstress your body, resulting in chronic fatigue, declining performance, and ultimately illness or injury. The effect of this mistake was demonstrated in a 2002 study conducted by researchers at the University of Birmingham and published in the *Journal of Applied Physiology*. Cyclists completed two weeks of normal training followed by two weeks of training in which their workload was doubled. Their time-trial performance was found to be 6.5 percent worse at the end of this block of intensified training than it had been after normal training.

Decreasing the training load from week to week: This causes an initial increase in performance capacity in fit individuals because it gives the body a chance to fully absorb the stress of recent training and overcome fatigue. This was shown in the final part of the Birmingham study I just described, where two weeks of sharply reduced training caused time-trial performance to rebound to a level that was 1.4 percent better than in the first time trial done after normal training. But prolonged decreases in training loads result in *detraining*, a reversal of the fitness-building process. For example, in a 1993 study, Danish researchers found that four weeks of sharply reduced training caused performance in an endurance test to drop by 21 percent in previously well-trained endurance athletes.

It is easy to avoid the negative consequences of all three alternatives to progressive overload with good planning. The following table offers an example of a sensible three-week pattern of progressive overload in the training of a generic athlete. (Note that the high-intensity training done on the first day of each week would necessarily be divided into short intervals.)

	Monday	Tuesday	Wednesday	Thursday	Friday	Saturday	Sunday
Week 1	40:00 with 24:00 at high intensity	40:00 at low intensity	40:00 at low intensity	40:00 with 24:00 at moderate intensity	40:00 at low intensity	1:00:00 at low intensity	Rest
Week 2	44:00 with 26:00 at high intensity	40:00 at low intensity	40:00 at low intensity	44:00 with 26:00 at moderate intensity	40:00 at low intensity	1:05:00 at low intensity	Rest
Week 3	48:00 with 28:00 at high intensity	40:00 at low intensity	40:00 at low intensity	48:00 with 28:00 at moderate intensity	40:00 at low intensity	1:10:00 at low intensity	Rest

If you're a noncompetitive exerciser rather than a competitive athlete, you need not practice progressive overload beyond the point where the training you're doing is yielding the benefits you seek. Thereafter you can choose to maintain a consistent routine, cutting back spontaneously for brief periods when your body needs a little extra rest and changing things up as much as you need to in order to keep from getting bored.

Purpose-Driven Workouts

If you knew absolutely nothing about how to prepare for races in your sport, your first intuition might be to just practice racing over and over—in other words, to make every workout a rehearsal for actual competition. This approach has been tried, and it hasn't worked very well. Generations of experimentation have revealed that racing performance is maximized when, instead of simulating competition in every workout, athletes work on individual components of endurance fitness separately in purpose-driven workouts.

In each endurance sport, there is a collection of tried-and-true standard workout types that all of the most successful racers do regularly. Some workouts focus on low intensity. Slow, steady sessions of short-to-moderate duration serve the purpose of developing and maintaining basic aerobic fitness and fat-burning capacity, while longer sessions at low intensity are used to increase raw endurance. Workouts focusing on moderate intensity often consist of an extended effort at moderate intensity sandwiched between an easy warm-up and a gentle cooldown (often called a "tempo" or "threshold" session). High-intensity training is almost always done in an interval format, with short, fast efforts separated by short periods of recovery at low intensity. In cycling and running, high-intensity intervals are often done on hills to add a strength-building element.

There are infinite permutations of each basic workout type, many of which are specific to individual sports. It is beyond the scope of this chapter to catalog all of them, nor is it necessary for you to learn and practice every single permutation that exists in your sport in order to maximize the results you get from the time and effort you invest in training. But it is important that you learn and practice all of the "bread-and-butter" workouts that are most commonly used to develop the various components of event-specific endurance fitness. Table 12.1 presents the full repertoire of bread-and-butter workouts in running. In my experience as a coach, at least one or two of these tools is missing from the typical recreational runner's purpose-driven workout toolbox.

Exercisers should not feel compelled to do all of the workouts that athletes do. The essential workouts for noncompetitive seekers of endurance fitness are easy runs or their equivalent in another activity and high-intensity intervals. These formats alone will enable you to adhere to the 80/20 Rule and reap its benefits. But it's okay to mix in other workouts if the variety helps sustain a high level of motivation for training.

Table 12.1 "Bread-and-Butter" Workouts for Runners

Workout Type	Description	Example	Variations
Easy Run	A short or relatively short run at a steady, low intensity	45:00 at a "conversational" pace	Recovery Run: An extraslow run done as the next run after a challenging workout Fast-Finish Run: An Easy Run finishing with a short effort at moderate intensity
Long Run	A prolonged run at a steady, low intensity	14 miles at a "conversational" pace	Marathon-Pace Run: A long run at marathon pace following an easy warm-up Long Fartlek Run: A long run featuring multiple, short surges at moderate to high intensity
Tempo Run	A steady effort at moderate intensity sandwiched between a warm-up and a cooldown	10:00 at a "conversational" pace 20:00 at half-marathon race pace 10:00 at a "conversational" pace	Cruise Intervals Run: A run featuring two to four efforts at moderate intensity, each lasting several minutes and separated by low-intensity active recoveries
Hill Repetitions Run	A run featuring multiple uphill efforts at high intensity separated by low-intensity active recoveries	10:00 at a "conversational" pace 10 x (1:00 uphill at high intensity/2:00 active recovery at low intensity) 10:00 at a "conversational" pace	Downhill Intervals Run: Structurally identical to a Hill Repetitions Run, but the high-intensity efforts are run downhill
High-Intensity Interval Run	A run featuring multiple efforts at high intensity, usually on a 400-meter track, separated by low-intensity active recoveries	10:00 at a "conversational" pace 6 x (800 meters at 5K race pace/2:00 active recovery at low intensity) 10:00 at a "conversational" pace	"New Intervals" Run: Structurally similar to a standard intervals run, but the active recoveries are performed at a faster pace to further challenge the body's capacity to recover quickly from acute fatigue

The Hard/Easy Rule

The Hard/Easy Rule states that the most challenging workouts an athlete does each week should be separated by one or more less-challenging workouts (or days of outright rest). For example, if you do three challenging workouts and three easier workouts in a given week, the challenging workouts should not fall on Monday, Tuesday, and Wednesday. Scheduling them on Monday, Wednesday, and Saturday would make more sense.

The Hard/Easy Rule exists because challenging workouts generate a significant amount of fatigue that takes time for the body to recover from. When challenging workouts are done too close together, fatigue becomes magnified to the point that it interferes with the body's fitness-boosting adaptations to training. In a 2014 study, Brazilian and American researchers found that subjects who performed exhaustive interval runs on three consecutive days exhibited signs of compromised immune function. This type of stress as well as others make challenging workouts less beneficial when performed consecutively than they would be if they were spread out over a slightly longer period of time.

Any training session that results in significant fatigue qualifies as challenging. This includes not only high-intensity interval workouts but also long workouts at low intensity. Generally, it is no more advisable to do a long endurance workout the day before or the day after an interval workout than it is to do back-to-back high-intensity interval workouts. Note that a rest day counts as an easy day, so it's okay to follow one challenging workout with another challenging workout if there's a rest day between them.

Select exceptions to the Hard/Easy Rule are allowable. For example, if you are preparing for a multiday stage race, you might want to perform challenging workouts on consecutive days occasionally to inure your body to the experience of pushing your limits when already fatigued from prior exercise.

The Hard/Easy Rule applies to exercisers and athletes equally. Whatever your goal is, doing back-to-back challenging workouts will make it harder for you to achieve.

Recovery Weeks

Fitness does not improve during workouts. It improves at rest, between workouts. Rest is therefore as important a part of the training process as exercise itself. Your body needs rest on three different timescales: micro, meso, and macro. The microscale is day to day, and we've just addressed it in our discussion of the Hard/Easy Rule. The macroscale encompasses the complete training cycle from the first day of base training through race day. I will discuss macroscale rest in the penultimate section of the chapter. Mesoscale rest occurs in the context of multiweek training blocks, each block concluding with a recovery week.

Recovery weeks work hand-in-hand with progressive overload. If you practice progressive overload, making each week of training a bit more challenging than your body is accustomed to, you will become increasingly fatigued, eventually reaching a point where your body is no longer benefiting from your hard work, unless you cut back periodically to give your body a chance to catch up on rest. Elite endurance athletes typically make every third or fourth week a recovery week.

The amount by which the training load is reduced in recovery weeks should depend on the context and on the individual athlete. A 30 percent reduction in total training time is a good place to start. In this scenario, if you exercise nine hours in the last week of hard training in a given block, you would aim to complete about six hours and 20 minutes of training in the recovery week that follows. The following week would then be slightly harder than the week that preceded the recovery week.

Exercisers who consistently maintain a training load that is easily managed do not need to plan recovery weeks. They should, however, cut back on training for a few days whenever unusual levels of fatigue or soreness indicate the need for extra rest.

Periodization

The term *periodization* refers to the practice of dividing the training process into distinct phases, each emphasizing a different type of training.

The classic approach to periodization begins with a base phase in which the athlete completes gradually increasing amounts of low-intensity training in order to gently develop the aerobic system, increase endurance, and enhance the body's ability to handle higher training loads. This is followed by a strength phase that serves to build a bridge between base training and speed training. The strength phase emphasizes high-intensity work against resistance: cycling or running uphill, swimming with handle paddles or fins, and so forth. After the strength phase comes a speed or intensity phase in which the most challenging workouts are done at race pace and faster. The final phase is a short taper phase, in which the training load is reduced stepwise to ensure the athlete is well-rested for competition.

Periodization is approached in somewhat different ways in different endurance disciplines and can even be done effectively in more than one way within a given sport. In recent years, for example, some elite cyclists have begun to experiment with an approach called *block periodization*, which entails separating the volume and intensity elements of training to some degree. For example, an athlete might do three high-intensity workouts and one low-intensity workout per week in every fourth week and do one high-intensity workout and three low-intensity workouts in other weeks.

Whether you choose the classic approach to periodization or the block approach, your training should become increasingly specific to the challenge of racing as your most important competition approaches. The types of training that are least similar to the race or races you're preparing for should be emphasized early in the training cycle and those that most closely simulate the specific demands of racing should dominate later in the training cycle.

Additionally, volume and intensity should be combined in such a way that the overall workload slowly increases as the training process unfolds. Typically, this is done by increasing volume while holding intensity steady in the early part of the training cycle and increasing intensity while holding volume steady (or even slightly decreasing volume) in the latter part.

There is no need whatsoever for exercisers to periodize their training. Periodization requires thoughtful planning, an effort that amounts to wasted time for those whose goal is to maintain the results they're already getting from their training.

Downtime

In our discussion of recovery weeks, I mentioned that seekers of endurance fitness require rest on three separate timescales. We've already discussed the first two: the microscale, where rest is obtained through observance of the Hard/Easy Rule, and the mesoscale, where rest is supplied by recovery weeks. The broadest timescale for rest is the macroscale, where rest is achieved through downtime, a multiweek period of sharply reduced training that falls between race-focused training cycles.

Just as recovery weeks are required because applying the Hard/Easy Rule does not provide enough rest to obviate the need for deeper rest on a broader timescale, downtime is needed because recovery weeks do not completely eliminate the need for an even deeper level of rest on an even broader timescale.

This important fact has been demonstrated in an interesting way by Stephen McGregor, an exercise physiologist at Eastern Michigan University and also a cycling coach. McGregor monitors the training of his athletes with the help of a software program called the Performance Management Chart (PMC), which quantifies fitness and fatigue levels through the input of training data. This tool is meant to be able to predict how well an individual athlete will perform in competition, and it does this quite well overall. However, McGregor has observed that when an athlete maintains a high level of fitness for an extended period time (usually four months or longer), performance tends to decline, even when fatigue is well managed and the PMC predicts improvement.

McGregor is not certain why this phenomenon occurs, but he suspects that prolonged hard training slowly fatigues the nervous system, so that the same training that increases performance initially causes it to decline later. Whatever the reason, highly competitive endurance athletes have long observed that heavy training offers diminishing returns over time until it becomes necessary to take a break and allow both body and mind to regenerate.

Elite athletes take downtime at least once and more often twice a year. In the most typical case, an athlete takes an extended break from structured training during the "off-season" period that begins after the last event of the competitive season and takes a shorter and/or less complete break roughly six months later. Off-season downtime might consist of two weeks with little or no exercise, whereas midseason downtime is more likely to consist of a couple of weeks of very light daily training. It seems that 24 weeks is about the maximum length of time that an athlete who is training for peak fitness can go without downtime.

Some athletes don't like taking downtime because it amounts to purposely giving away hard-earned fitness. But sacrificing current fitness in this way creates the opportunity to attain a higher level of fitness in the long term. When you begin a new training cycle after downtime, you will be fresher than you were at the end of your last training cycle yet fitter than you were at the start of that cycle. As a result, you will be fitter than ever at the end of the new cycle.

Noncompetitive exercisers who maintain consistent, moderate training loads seldom require downtime. The challenge for many exercisers is avoiding unplanned and unneeded downtime as a consequence of low motivation. One way exercisers can escape this problem is to become athletes. Preparing for races is powerfully motivating and has a way of drawing fitness seekers into a seasonal routine in which breaks from exercise become a helpful part of the overall plan rather than harmful interruptions to the plan. If you decide to go down this road, you'll want to begin following athlete guidelines for all eight essential training methods, not just periodization.

Strength Training

To perform optimally in races, rowers need to do more than row, swimmers need to do more than swim, and cross-country skiers need to do more than ski. All of these types of endurance athlete and others must supplement their sport-specific training with strength training in order to attain true peak performance in competition.

Studies prove it. In 2011, researchers at the Norwegian School of Sport Science reported that twelve weeks of supplemental strength training improved double-poling performance in a group of elite junior cross-country skiers. Four years later, a study conducted by scientists at the University of Greenwich and published in the *International Journal of Physiology and Performance* found that recreational runners who completed six weeks of supplemental strength training experienced a 3.6 percent improvement in 5K race times. Similar results have come out of studies involving other types of endurance athletes.

Strength training is also believed to reduce injury risk in endurance athletes, although there is little scientific proof of this. Research has shown, however, that weakness in particular muscles predisposes certain types of athlete to injury. For example, runners with weak hip abductors and hip external rotators are more likely to develop overuse injuries of the knee. It stands to reason that strengthening these muscles would reduce the risk for this type of injury.

There are many ways to strength train and not all of them are equally beneficial to endurance athletes. An effective program will include movements that condition the so-called prime movers, or larger muscles that do the most work in a given activity. It is helpful to develop not only the strength of these muscles but also their fatigue resistance. Strength-building requires heavy loads, whereas muscular endurance comes from lighter loads and higher reps. Exercise selection is important as well. It is best to condition the prime movers with functional exercises that mimic aspects of sports movements rather than with isolation exercises like the ones that bodybuilders favor. For example, cyclists are better off strengthening the quadriceps muscles on the front of the thigh with bench step-ups than with machine leg extensions.

An effective strength-training program will also include exercises targeting smaller muscles that play important balancing or stabilizing roles during sports movements. The small muscles of the rotator cuff play such a role in swimmers. These muscles tend to be relatively weak compared to the highly developed prime movers of the chest and upper back, but giving them due attention in the gym will reduce the risk for the shoulder injuries that are so common in swimmers.

A little strength training goes a long way. Some studies have shown that as few as two half-hour sessions per week yield significant results. As an endurance athlete, you want to avoid doing more strength training than is necessary so that fatigue produced by these sessions doesn't interfere with your sport-specific training.

Strength training is advisable for exercisers as well as athletes, but for a different reason. Although the performance benefits of strength training are not relevant to exercisers, and although exercisers are less prone to the overuse injuries that a good strength-training program may help prevent, strength training complements endurance training with respect to the goal of developing a leaner body composition.

If getting leaner is your top priority, you'll want to select different exercises than you would if competitive performance was the main objective. Traditional movements like bench presses that do little for athletes carry the benefit of building more muscle mass, which in turn increases resting metabolism and ultimately burns more fat than many of the functional movements that are most beneficial to racers.

Follow the Leaders

There isn't enough room in this book to supply all of the guidance needed to train effectively in every endurance discipline. But I trust that I have made the point that you will get the best results from your training if you emulate the methods used by elite endurance athletes, just as you will get the greatest possible benefit from your diet if you eat like the world's fittest people.

In my work as a running and triathlon coach as well as a sports nutritionist, I take great satisfaction in seeing the breakthroughs that occur when an athlete or exerciser begins to train or eat like the pros.

As you might expect, the greatest breakthroughs occur in those who do both. Take Holly, a physician and runner in her forties from Kansas, who after twelve years of "winging" her training and diet and making little progress began to follow an "80/20" training plan I created, to cook Georgie Fear's recipes (Holly actually served as a tester for the recipes in this book), and to track her Diet Quality Score. In just two months she lost 6 pounds and 2 percent body fat and bettered her 5K race time by a full minute. What's more, she enjoyed both her running and her eating more than ever before.

What works for the world's fittest people worked for Holly, and what worked for Holly will work for you. Will the next breakthrough be yours?

APPENDIX A
A PERFECT DAY SAMPLE TABLE

Use this table according to the guidelines described in Chapter 8 to create your Endurance Diet Perfect Day.

Current Routine	Things to Improve	Features to Retain	Perfect Day
Breakfast (TIME)			
Snack (TIME)			
Lunch (TIME)			
Snack (TIME)			
Dinner (TIME)			
Snack (TIME)			

ACKNOWLEDGMENTS

I COULD NOT HAVE WRITTEN THIS BOOK WITHOUT THE GENEROUS HELP OF the dozens of athletes who willing shared detailed information about their diets and, in many cases, allowed me to eat and even train with them. Although many of these athletes are named within the book, a great many others are not but their contributions are no less valuable. I am extremely grateful also to the coaches, nutritionists, and others who served as conduits to these athletes, especially Marina Bonilha, Arseny Chernov, Louis Delajaije, Nobuya Hashizume, Anna Novick, Cory Nyamora, Pete Pfitzinger, Marco Pinotti, and Justin Wadsworth. Other valuable contributions were made by Brandon Bauer, Kate Buntenbach, Jeffrey Gopsill, Lori Henderson, Tom Hood, Asker Jeukendrup, Mike Kane, Patrick McKenna, Ruben Orduz, Stephanie Riis, Marcella Shandor, Trent Stellingwerff, Patti Thompson, Holly Winchell, Jordan Zwick, and Renee Sedliar and the rest of the great team at Da Capo Lifelong Books. Thank you all!

REFERENCES

Chapter 1

Ciccolo JT, Bartholomew JB, Stults-Kolehmainen M, Seifert J, Portman R. 2009. Relationship between body weight and health-related quality of life amongst a large group of highly active individuals. Paper presented at the Society for Behavioral Medicine, Montreal, Canada.

Seiler KS, Kjerland GØ. Quantifying training intensity distribution in elite endurance athletes: is there evidence for an "optimal" distribution? *Scand J Med Sci Sports.* 2006 Feb;16(1):49-56.

Chapter 2

Bouchard C. Genomic predictors of trainability. *Experimental Physiology.* 97:347-352. doi:10.1113/expphysiol.2011.058735.

Jarvis M, McNaughton L, Seddon A, Thompson D. The acute 1-week effects of the Zone diet on body composition, blood lipid levels, and performance in recreational endurance athletes. *J Strength Cond Res.* 2002 Feb;16(1):50-7.

Legaz-Arrese A, Kinfu H, Munguía-Izquierdo D, Carranza-Garcia LE, Calderón FJ. Basic physiological measures determine fitness and are associated with running performance in elite young male and female Ethiopian runners. *J Sports Med Phys Fitness.* 2009 Dec;49(4):358-63.

Mayfield J. *The Engine of Complexity.* New York, NY: Columbia University Press; 2013, 149.

Mitsuishi M, Miyashita K, Muraki A, Tamaki M, Tanaka K, Itoh H. Dietary protein decreases exercise endurance through rapamycin-sensitive suppression of muscle mitochondria. *Am J Physiol Endocrinol Metab.* 2013 Oct 1;305(7):E776-84.

Muñoz I, Seiler S, Bautista J, España J, Larumbe E, Esteve-Lanao. Does polarized training improve performance in recreational runners? *J Int J Sports Physiol Perform.* 2014 Mar;9(2):265-72.

Rehm CD, Peñalvo JL, Afshin A, Mozaffarian D. Dietary intake among US Adults, 1999-2012. *JAMA.* 2016 Jun 21;315(23):2542-53. doi:10.1001/jama.2016.7491.

Romero P, Wagg J, Green M, Kaiser D, Krummenacker M, Karp P. Computational prediction of human metabolic pathways from the complete human genome. *Genome Biol.* 2005;6(1):R2.

Sears B, with Lawren B. *Enter the Zone* New York, NY: Regan Books; 1995, ix.

257

Chapter 3

Addessi E, Mancini A, Crescimbene L, Ariely D and Visalberghi E. How to spend a token? Trade-offs between food variety and food preference in tufted capuchin monkeys (*Cebus apella*). *Behavioural Processes*. 2010;83(3):267.

Cerling TE, Manthi FK, Mbua EN, Leakey LN, Leakey MG, Leakey RE, Brown FH, Grine FE, Hart JA, Kaleme P, Roche H, Uno KT, Wood BA. Stable isotope-based diet reconstructions of Turkana Basin hominins. *Proc Natl Acad Sci USA*. 2013 Jun 25;110(26):10501-6.

Gavaghan J. Hooked on chicken nuggets: girl, 17, who has eaten nothing else since age TWO rushed to hospital after collapsing. DailyMail.com. http://www.dailymail.co.uk/health/article-2092071/Stacey-Irvine-17-collapses-eating-McDonalds-chicken-nuggets-age-2.html. Accessed February 14, 2015.

Krebs-Smith SM, Smiciklas-Wright H, Guthrie HA, Krebs-Smith J. The effects of variety in food choices on dietary quality. *J Am Diet Assoc*. 1987 Jul;87(7):897-903.

Kuijer RG, Boyce JA, Marshall EM. Associating a prototypical forbidden food item with guilt or celebration: relationships with indicators of (un)healthy eating and the moderating role of stress and depressive symptoms. *Psychol Health*. 2015;30(2):203-17.

Mirmiran P, Azadbakht L, Azizi F. Dietary diversity within food groups: an indicator of specific nutrient adequacy in Tehranian women. *J Am Coll Nutr*. 2006 Aug;25(4):354-61.

Murphy SP, Foote JA, Wilkens LR, Basiotis PP, Carlson A, White KK, Yonemori KM. Simple measures of dietary variety are associated with improved dietary quality. *J Am Diet Assoc*. 2006 Mar;106(3):425-9.

Reedy J, Krebs-Smith SM, Miller PE, Liese AD, Kahle LL, Park Y, Subar AF. Higher diet quality is associated with decreased risk of all-cause, cardiovascular disease, and cancer mortality among older adults. *J Nutr*. 2014 Jun;144(6):881-9. doi:10.3945/jn.113.189407. Epub 2014 Feb 26.

Schwerin HS, Stanton JL, Smith JL, Riley AM Jr, Brett BE. Food, eating habits, and health: a further examination of the relationship between food eating patterns and nutritional health. *Am J Clin Nutr*. 1982 May;35(5 Suppl):1319-25.

Slattery ML. Defining dietary consumption: is the sum greater than its parts? *Am J Clin Nutr*. 2008 July;88(1):14-15.

Stubbs RJ, Johnstone AM, Mazlan N, Mbaiwa SE, Ferris S. Effect of altering the variety of sensorially distinct foods, of the same macronutrient content, on food intake and body weight in men. *Eur J Clin Nutr*. 2001 Jan;55(1):19-28.

Zampollo F, Kniffin KM, Wansink B, Shimizu M. Food plating preferences of children: the importance of presentation on desire for diversity. *Acta Paediatrica*. 2012;101:61-66.

Chapter 4

Alkerwi A. Diet quality concept. *Nutrition*. 2014 Jun;30(6):613-8.

Bennett H. Dispatch: Fernanda Keller – Style Smile and Soul. *Triathlete*. http://triathlon.competitor.com/2012/12/features/dispatch-fernanda-keller-style-smiles-and-soul_67366. Accessed April 9, 2015.

Boada LD, Henríquez-Hernández LA, Luzardo OP. The impact of red and processed meat consumption on cancer and other health outcomes: epidemiological evidences. *Food Chem Toxicol*. 2016 Jun;92:236-44. doi:10.1016/j.fct.2016.04.008. Epub 2016 Apr 20. Review.

Ericson U, Hellstrand S, Brunkwall L, Schulz CA, Sonestedt E, Wallström P, Gullberg B, Wirfält E, Orho-Melander M. Food sources of fat may clarify the inconsistent role of dietary fat intake for incidence of type 2 diabetes. *Am J Clin Nutr*. 2015 May;101(5):1065-80.

Firląg M, Kamaszewski M, Adamek D, Gajewska M, Bałasińska B. Long-term consumption of fish oil partially protects brain tissue from age-related neurodegeneration. *Postepy Hig Med Dosw* (Online). 2015 Feb 6;69:188-96.

Fung TT, Hu FB, Pereira MA, Liu S, Stampfer MJ, Colditz GA, Willett WC. Whole-grain intake and the risk of type 2 diabetes: a prospective study in men. *Am J Clin Nutr*. 2002 Sep;76(3):535-40.

Giacco R, Costabile G, Della Pepa G, Anniballi G, Griffo E, Mangione A, Cipriano P, Viscovo D, Clemente G, Landberg R, Pacini G, Rivellese AA, Riccardi G. A whole-grain cereal-based diet lowers postprandial plasma insulin and triglyceride levels in individuals with metabolic syndrome. *Nutr Metab Cardiovasc Dis*. 2014 Aug;24(8): 837-44.

Kanda A, Nakayama K, Sanbongi C, Nagata M, Ikegami S, Itoh H. Effects of Whey, Caseinate, or Milk Protein Ingestion on Muscle Protein Synthesis after Exercise. Nutrients. 2016 Jun 3;8(6). pii: E339. doi:10.3390/nu8060339.

Katcher HI, Legro RS, Kunselman AR, Gillies PJ, Demers LM, Bagshaw DM, Kris-Etherton PM. The effects of a whole grain-enriched hypocaloric diet on cardiovascular disease risk factors in men and women with metabolic syndrome. *Am J Clin Nutr*. 2008 Jan;87(1):79-90.

Kim H, Park S, Yang H, Choi YJ, Huh KB, Chang N. Association between fish and shellfish, and omega-3 PUFAs intake and CVD risk factors in middle-aged female patients with type 2 diabetes. *Nutr Res Pract*. 2015 Oct;9(5):496-502. doi:10.4162/nrp.2015.9.5.496. Epub 2015 May 13.

McKeown NM, Troy LM, Jacques PF, Hoffmann U, O'Donnell CJ, Fox CS. Whole- and refined-grain intakes are differentially associated with abdominal visceral and subcutaneous adiposity in healthy adults: the Framingham Heart Study. *Am J Clin Nutr*. 2010 Nov;92(5):1165-71.

Mozaffarian D, Hao T, Rimm EB, Willett WC, Hu FB. Changes in diet and lifestyle and long-term weight gain in women and men. *N Engl J Med*. 2011 Jun 23;364(25):2392-404.

Mozaffarian D, Kumanyika SK, Lemaitre RN, Olson JL, Burke GL, Siscovick DS. Cereal, fruit, and vegetable fiber intake and the risk of cardiovascular disease in elderly individuals. *JAMA*. 2003 Apr 2;289(13):1659-66.

Musumeci G, Maria Trovato F, Imbesi R, Castrogiovanni P. Effects of dietary extra-virgin olive oil on oxidative stress resulting from exhaustive exercise in rat skeletal muscle: a morphological study. *Acta Histochem*. 2014 Jan;116(1):61-9.

Randolph JM, Edirisinghe I, Masoni AM, Kappagoda T, Burton-Freeman B. Potatoes, glycemic index, and weight loss in free-living individuals: practical implications. *J Am Coll Nutr*. 2014;33(5):375-84.

Rohrmann S1, Overvad K, Bueno-de-Mesquita HB, Jakobsen MU, Egeberg R, Tjønneland A, Nailler L, Boutron-Ruault MC, Clavel-Chapelon F, Krogh V, Palli D, Panico S, Tumino R, Ricceri F, Bergmann MM, Boeing H, Li K, Kaaks R, Khaw KT, Wareham NJ, Crowe FL, Key TJ, Naska A, Trichopoulou A, Trichopoulos D, Leenders M, Peeters PH, Engeset D, Parr CL, Skeie G, Jakszyn P, Sánchez MJ, Huerta JM, Redondo ML, Barricarte A, Amiano P, Drake I, Sonestedt E, Hallmans G, Johansson I, Fedirko V, Romieux I, Ferrari P, Norat T, Vergnaud AC, Riboli E, Linseisen J. Meat consumption and mortality—results from the European Prospective Investigation into Cancer and Nutrition. BMC Med. 2013 Mar 7;11:63.

Rondini R. Frenanda Keller Triathlon. Magazine SuperAção. https://translate.google.com /translate?hl=en&sl=pt&u=http://www.webrun.com.br/h/noticias/fernanda-triath lon-keller/1507&prev=search. Accessed August 9, 2016.

Rowan, Karen. Big fat disconnect: 90% of us think our diets are healthy. Live Science. http://www.livescience.com/10389-big-fat-disconnect-90-diets-healthy.html. Accessed May 20, 2015.

Wang X, Ouyang Y, Liu J, Zhu M, Zhao G, Bao W, Hu FB. Fruit and vegetable consumption and mortality from all causes, cardiovascular disease, and cancer: systematic review and dose-response meta-analysis of prospective cohort studies. BMJ. 2014 Jul 29;349:g4490. doi:10.1136/bmj.g4490.

Watson TA, Callister R, Taylor RD, Sibbritt DW, MacDonald-Wicks LK, Garg ML. Antioxidant restriction and oxidative stress in short-duration exhaustive exercise. Med Sci Sports Exerc. 2005 Jan;37(1):63-71.

Yang Q, Zhang Z, Gregg EW, Flanders WD, Merritt R, Hu FB. Added sugar intake and cardiovascular diseases mortality among US adults. JAMA Intern Med. 2014 Apr;174(4):516-24.

Żebrowska A, Mizia-Stec K, Mizia M, Gąsior Z, Poprzęcki S. Omega-3 fatty acids supplementation improves endothelial function and maximal oxygen uptake in endurance-trained athletes. Eur J Sport Sci. 2015;15(4):305-14.

Zhang X, Shu XO, Xiang YB, Yang G, Li H, Gao J, Cai H, Gao YT, Zheng W. Cruciferous vegetable consumption is associated with a reduced risk of total and cardiovascular disease mortality. Am J Clin Nutr. 2011 Jul;94(1):240-6.

Chapter 5

Achten J, Halson SL, Moseley L, Rayson MP, Casey A, Jeukendrup AE. Higher dietary carbohydrate content during intensified running training results in better maintenance of performance and mood state. J Appl Physiol (1985). 2004 Apr;96(4):1331-40.

AlEssa HB, Bhupathiraju SN, Malik VS, Wedick NM, Campos H, Rosner B, Willett WC, Hu FB. Carbohydrate quality and quantity and risk of type 2 diabetes in US women. Am J Clin Nutr. 2015 Dec;102(6):1543-53.

Badenhorst CE, Dawson B, Cox GR, Laarakkers CM, Swinkels DW, Peeling P. Acute dietary carbohydrate manipulation and the subsequent inflammatory and hepcidin responses to exercise. Eur J Appl Physiol. 2015 Dec;115(12):2521-30.

Bisschop PH, de Metz J, Ackermans MT, Endert E, Pijl H, Kuipers F, Meijer AJ, Sauerwein HP, Romijn JA. Dietary fat content alters insulin-mediated glucose metabolism in healthy men. *Am J Clin Nutr.* 2001 Mar;73(3):554-9.

Burke LM, Cox GR, Culmmings NK, Desbrow B. Guidelines for daily carbohydrate intake: do athletes achieve them? *Sports Med.* 2001;31(4):267-99.

Carlsohn A, Nippe S, Heydenreich J, Mayer F. Carbohydrate intake and food sources of junior triathletes during a moderate and an intensive training period. *Int J Sport Nutr Exerc Metab.* 2012 Dec;22(6):438-43.

Frentsos JA, Baer JT. Increased energy and nutrient intake during training and competition improves elite triathletes' endurance performance. *Int J Sport Nutr.* 1997 Mar;7(1):61-71.

Grossman SP. The role of glucose, insulin and glucagon in the regulation of food intake and body weight. *Neurosci Biobehav Rev.* 1986 Fall;10(3):295-315.

Hall KD, Bemis T, Brychta R, Chen KY, Courville A, Crayner EJ, Goodwin S, Guo J, Howard L, Knuth ND, Miller BV 3rd, Prado CM, Siervo M, Skarulis MC, Walter M, Walter PJ, Yannai L. Calorie for calorie, dietary fat restriction results in more body fat loss than carbohydrate restriction in people with obesity. *Cell Metab.* 2015 Sep 1;22(3):427-36.

Hill JO, Peters JC, Reed GW, Schlundt DG, Sharp T, Greene HL. Nutrient balance in humans: effects of diet composition. *Am J Clin Nutr.* 1991 Jul;54(1):10-7.

Lippi G, Salvagno GL, Danese E, Tarperi C, La Torre A, Guidi GC, Schena F. The baseline serum value of α-amylase is a significant predictor of distance running performance. *Clin Chem Lab Med.* 2015 Feb;53(3):469-76.

McCarthy J. Americans more likely to avoid drinking soda than before. Gallup.com. http://www.gallup.com/poll/174137/americans-likely-avoid-drinking-soda.aspx. Accessed July 14, 2015.

McEvoy CT, Cardwell CR, Woodside JV, Young IS, Hunter SJ, McKinley MC. A posteriori dietary patterns are related to risk of type 2 diabetes: findings from a systematic review and meta-analysis. *J Acad Nutr Diet.* 2014 Nov;114(11):1759-75.e4.

Neumark-Sztainer D, Wall M, Guo J, Story M, Haines J, Eisenberg M. Obesity, disordered eating, and eating disorders in a longitudinal study of adolescents: how do dieters fare 5 years later? *J Am Diet Assoc.* 2006 Apr;106(4):559-68.

Nielsen SJ, Popkin BM. Patterns and trends in food portion sizes, 1977-1998. *JAMA.* 2003 Jan 22-29;289(4):450-3.

Onywera VO, Kiplamai FK, Boit MK, Pitsiladis YP. Food and macronutrient intake of elite kenyan distance runners. *Int J Sport Nutr Exerc Metab.* 2004 Dec;14(6):709-19.

Romon M, Lebel P, Velly C, Marecaux N, Fruchart JC, Dallongeville J. Leptin response to carbohydrate or fat meal and association with subsequent satiety and energy intake. *Am J Physiol.* 1999 Nov;277(5 Pt 1):E855-61.

Schulte EM, Avena NM, Gearhardt AN. Which foods may be addictive? The roles of processing, fat content, and glycemic load. *PLoS One.* 2015 Feb 18;10(2):e0117959.

Sichieri R, Moura AS, Genelhu V, Hu F, Willett WC. An 18-mo randomized trial of a low-glycemic-index diet and weight change in Brazilian women. *Am J Clin Nutr.* 2007 Sep;86(3):707-13.

Turner-McGrievy GM, Davidson CR, Wingard EE, Wilcox S, Frongillo EA. Comparative effectiveness of plant-based diets for weight loss: a randomized controlled trial of five different diets. *Nutrition*. 2015 Feb;31(2):350-8.

Zajac A, Poprzecki S, Maszczyk A, Czuba M, Michalczyk M, Zydek G. The effects of a ketogenic diet on exercise metabolism and physical performance in off-road cyclists. *Nutrients*. 2014 Jun 27;6(7):2493-508.

Chapter 6

American Institute for Cancer Research. As restaurant portions grow, vast majority of Americans still belong to the clean plate club. Charitywire.com. http://www.charity wire.com/charity10/00235.html. Accessed August 30, 2015.

Artins C, Morgan L, Truby H. A review of the effects of exercise on appetite regulation: an obesity perspective. *International Journal of Obesity*. 2008;32:1337–1347. doi:10.1038/ijo.2008.98.

Barrack MT, Rauh MJ, Barkai HS, Nichols JF. Dietary restraint and low bone mass in female adolescent endurance runners. *Am J Clin Nutr*. 2008 Jan;87(1):36-43.

Brown AJ, Smith LT, Craighead LW. Appetite awareness as a mediator in an eating disorders prevention program. *Eat Disord*. 2010 Jul-Aug;18(4):286-301.

Buckner AL. Appetite awareness training in the prevention of eating disorders. Unpublished doctoral thesis. http://search.proquest.com/docview/304888376. 2008 Jan.

Cava E, Fontana L. Will calorie restriction work in humans? *Aging*. 2013 Jul;5(7):507-14.

Ciampolini M, Lovell-Smith D, Sifone M. Sustained self-regulation of energy intake. Loss of weight in overweight subjects. Maintenance of weight in normal-weight subjects. *Nutr Metab* (Lond). 2010 Jan 19;7:4.

Ciccolo JT, Bartholomew JB, Stults-Kolehmainen M, Seifert J, Portman R. 2009. Relationship between body weight and health-related quality of life amongst a large group of highly active individuals. Paper presented at the Society for Behavioral Medicine, Montreal, Canada.

Fothergill E, Guo J, Howard L, Kerns JC, Knuth ND, Brychta R, Chen KY, Skarulis MC, Walter M, Walter PJ, Hall KD. Persistent metabolic adaptation 6 years after "The Biggest Loser" competition. *Obesity*. 2016 Aug;24(8):1612-9. doi:10.1002/oby.21538. Epub 2016 May 2.

Fox MK, Devaney B, Reidy K, Razafindrakoto C, Ziegler P. Relationship between portion size and energy intake among infants and toddlers: evidence of self-regulation. *J Am Diet Assoc*. 2006 Jan;106(1 Suppl 1):S77-83.

Friedlaender JS, Rhoads JG. Patterns of adult weight and fat change in six Solomon Islands societies: a semi-longitudinal study. *Soc Sci Med*. 1982;16(2):205-15.

Harris JL, Bargh JA, Brownell KD. Priming effects of television food advertising on eating behavior. *Health psychol*. 2009 July;28(4):404-413.

Melin A, Tornberg AB, Skouby S, Møller SS, Sundgot-Borgen J, Faber J, Sidelmann JJ, Aziz M, Sjödin A. Energy availability and the female athlete triad in elite endurance athletes. *Scand J Med Sci Sports*. 2014 May 30.

Patton GC, Johnson-Sabine E, Wood K, Mann AH, Wakeling A. Abnormal eating attitudes in London schoolgirls—a prospective epidemiological study: outcome at twelve month follow-up. *Psychol Med.* 1990 May;20(2):383-94.

Silva JR. Overeating and restrained eaters: an affective neuroscience perspective. *Rev Med Chil.* 2008 Oct;136(10):1336-42.

Veenstra EM, de Jong PJ. Restrained eaters show enhanced automatic approach tendencies towards food. *Appetite.* 2010 Aug;55(1):30-6. *Rev Med Chil.* 2008 Oct;136(10): 1336-42.

Wansink B. *Mindless Eating.* New York, NY: Random House; 2006.

Waugh EJ, Polivy J, Ridout R, Hawker GA. A prospective investigation of the relations among cognitive dietary restraint, subclinical ovulatory disturbances, physical activity, and bone mass in healthy young women. *Am J Clin Nutr.* 2007 Dec;86(6):1791-801.

Young LR, Nestle M. The contribution of expanding portion sizes to the US obesity epidemic. *Am J Public Health.* 2002 Feb;92(2):246-249.

Chapter 7

Biesiekierski JR, Peters SL, Newnham ED, Rosella O, Muir JG, Gibson PR. No effects of gluten in patients with self-reported non-celiac gluten sensitivity following dietary reduction of low-fermentable, poorly-absorbed, short-chain carbohydrates. *Gastroenterology.* 2013 May 3;pii: S0016-5085(13)00702-6.

Fitzgerald M, Fear G. *Racing Weight Cookbook.* Boulder, CO: VeloPress; 2013.

Knibb RC, Armstrong A, Booth DA, Platts RG, Booth IW, MacDonald A. Psychological characteristics of people with perceived food intolerance in a community sample. *J Psychosom Res.* 1999 Dec;47(6):545-54.

Porcari J, Foster C. Mind Over Body. *ACE FitnessMatters.* May/June 2006.

Qi Q, Xu M, Wu H, Liang L, Champagne CM, Bray GA, Sacks FM, Qi L. IRS1 genotype modulates metabolic syndrome reversion in response to 2-year weight-loss diet intervention: the POUNDS LOST trial. *Diabetes Care.* 2013 Nov;36(11):3442-7.

Scheibehenne B, Miesler L, Todd PM. Fast and frugal food choices: uncovering individual decision heuristics. *Appetite.* 2007 Nov;49(3):578-89.

www.foodnavigator.com/Science/Health-and-nutrition-labels-may-have-negative-impact -on-taste-expectation-Study.

Chapter 8

Barnes TD, Kubota Y, Hu D, Jin DZ, Graybiel AM. Activity of striatal neurons reflects dynamic encoding and recoding of procedural memories. *Nature.* 2005 Oct 20; 437(7062):1158-61.

Deckersbach T, Das SK, Urban LE, Salinardi T, Batra P, Rodman AM, Arulpragasam AR, Dougherty DD, Roberts SB. Pilot randomized trial demonstrating reversal of obesity-related abnormalities in reward system responsivity to food cues with a behavioral intervention. *Nutr Diabetes.* 2014 Sep 1;4:e129.

Duhigg C. *The Power of Habit: Why We Do What We Do in Life and Business*. New York, NY: Random House; 2012.

Finch EA, Linde JA, Jeffery RW, Rothman AJ, King CM, Levy RL. The effects of outcome expectations and satisfaction on weight loss and maintenance: correlational and experimental analyses—a randomized trial. *Health Psychol*. 2005 Nov;24(6):608-16.

Neal DT, Wood W, Drolet A. How do people adhere to goals when willpower is low? The profits (and pitfalls) of strong habits. *J Pers and Soc Psychol*. 2013 Jun;104(6):959-75. doi:10.1037/a0032626.

Prinsen S, de Ridder DT, de Vet E. Eating by example: effects of environmental cues on dietary decisions. *Appetite*. 2013 Nov;70:1-5.

Robinson E, Higgs S. Food choices in the presence of 'healthy' and 'unhealthy' eating partners. *Br J Nutr*. 2013 Feb 28;109(4):765-71.

van de Giessen E, la Fleur SE, Eggels L, de Bruin K, van den Brink W, Booij J. High fat/carbohydrate ratio but not total energy intake induces lower striatal dopamine D2/3 receptor availability in diet-induced obesity. *Int J Obes* (Lond). 2013 May;37(5):754-7. doi: 10.1038/ijo.2012.128. Epub 2012 Aug 7.

Chapter 9

Ballor DL, Katch VL, Becque MD, Marcks CR. Resistance weight training during caloric restriction enhances lean body weight maintenance. *Am J Clin Nutr*. 1988 Jan;47(1):19-25.

Bray GA, Redman LM, de Jonge L, Covington J, Rood J, Brock C, Mancuso S, Martin CK, Smith SR. Effect of protein overfeeding on energy expenditure measured in a metabolic chamber. *Am J Clin Nutr*. 2015 Mar;101(3):496-505.

Dellavalle DM, Haas JD. Iron status is associated with endurance performance and training in female rowers. *Med Sci Sports Exerc*. 2012 Aug;44(8):1552-9.

Durrant ML, Garrow JS, Royston P, et al. Factors influencing the composition of the weight lost by obese patients on a reducing diet. *British Journal of Nutrition*. 1980;44(3):275-285.

Jeukendrup A, Brouns F, Wagenmakers AJ, Saris WH. Carbohydrate-electrolyte feedings improve 1 h time trial cycling performance. *Int J Sports Med*. 1997 Feb;18(2):125-9.

Jeukendrup AE, Hopkins S, Aragón-Vargas LF, Hulston C. No effect of carbohydrate feeding on 16 km cycling time trial performance. *Eur J Appl Physiol*. 2008 Nov;104(5):831-7. doi: 10.1007/s00421-008-0838-z. Epub 2008 Sep 24.

King AC, Castro CM, Buman MP, Hekler EB, Urizar GG Jr, Ahn DK. Behavioral impacts of sequentially versus simultaneously delivered dietary plus physical activity interventions: the CALM trial. *Ann Behav Med*. 2013 Oct;46(2):157-68.

Lewis EJ, Radonic PW, Wolever TM, Wells GD. 21 days of mammalian omega-3 fatty acid supplementation improves aspects of neuromuscular function and performance in male athletes compared to olive oil placebo. *J Int Soc Sports Nutr*. 2015 Jun 18;12:28.

Lunn, WR, Finn JA, Axtell RS. Effects of sprint interval training and body weight reduction on power to weight ratio in experienced cyclists. *J Strength Cond Res*. 2009 23(4):1217-24.

Marquet LA, Brisswalter J, Louis J, Tiollier E, Burke LM, Hawley JA, Hausswirth C. Enhanced endurance performance by periodization of carbohydrate intake: "Sleep Low" strategy. *Med Sci Sports Exerc.* 2016 Apr;48(4):663-72. doi:10.1249/MSS.0000000000000823.

Mettler S, Zimmermann MB. Iron excess in recreational marathon runners. *Eur J Clin Nutr.* 2010 May;64(5):490-4.

Nehlsen-Cannarella SL, Fagoaga OR, Nieman DC, Henson DA, Butterworth DE, Schmitt RL, Bailey EM, Warren BJ, Utter A, Davis JM. Carbohydrate and the cytokine response to 2.5 h of running. *J Appl Physiol* (1985). 1997 May;82(5):1662-7.

Papanikolaou Y, Brooks J, Reider C, Fulgoni VL 3rd. US adults are not meeting recommended levels for fish and omega-3 fatty acid intake: results of an analysis using observational data from NHANES 2003-2008. *Nutr J.* 2014 Apr 2;13:31.

Psilander N, Frank P, Flockhart M, Sahlin K. Exercise with low glycogen increases PGC-1α gene expression in human skeletal muscle. *Eur J Appl Physiol.* 2013 Apr;113(4):951-63. doi:10.1007/s00421-012-2504-8. Epub 2012 Oct 2.

Snyder AC, Dvorak LL, Roepke JB. Influence of dietary iron source on measures of iron status among female runners. *Med Sci Sports Exerc.* 1989 Feb;21(1):7-10.

Weigle DS, Breen PA, Matthys CC, Callahan HS, Meeuws KE, Burden VR, Purnell JQ. A high-protein diet induces sustained reductions in appetite, ad libitum caloric intake, and body weight despite compensatory changes in diurnal plasma leptin and ghrelin concentrations. *Am J Clin Nutr.* 2005 Jul;82(1):41-8.

Willis KS, Smith DT, Broughton KS, Larson-Meyer DE. Vitamin D status and biomarkers of inflammation in runners. *Open Access J Sports Med.* 2012 Apr 27;3:35-42.

Chapter 10

Alaunyte I, Stojceska V, Plunkett A, Derbyshire E. Dietary iron intervention using a staple food product for improvement of iron status in female runners. *J Int Soc Sports Nutr.* 2014 Oct 18;11(1):50. doi:10.1186/s12970-014-0050-y. eCollection 2014.

Bell PG, Walshe IH, Davison GW, Stevenson E, Howatson G. Montmorency cherries reduce the oxidative stress and inflammatory responses to repeated days high-intensity stochastic cycling. *Nutrients.* 2014 Feb 21;6(2):829-43.

Clayton D. *Running to the Top.* Mountain View, CA: Anderson World; 1980, 16.

Del Coso J, Muñoz G, Muñoz-Guerra J. Prevalence of caffeine use in elite athletes following its removal from the World Anti-Doping Agency list of banned substances. *Appl Physiol Nutr Metab.* 2011 Aug;36(4):555-61.

Drewnowski A. New metrics of affordable nutrition: which vegetables provide most nutrients for least cost? *J Acad Nutr Diet.* 2013 Sep;113(9):1182-7.

Geliebter A, Lee MI, Abdillahi M, Jones J. Satiety following intake of potatoes and other carbohydrate test meals. *Ann Nutr Metab.* 2013;62(1):37-43.

Habte K, Adish A, Zerfu D, Kebede A, Moges D, Tesfaye D, Challa F, Baye K. Iron, folate and vitamin B$_{12}$ status of Ethiopian professional runners. *Nutr Metab* (Lond). 2015 Dec 30;12:62. doi:10.1186/s12986-015-0056-8. eCollection 2015.

Harms-Ringdahl M, Jenssen D, Haghdoost S. Tomato juice intake suppressed serum concentration of 8-oxodG after extensive physical activity. *Nutr J.* 2012 May 2;11:29.

Hart N, Sarga L, Csende Z, Koltai E, Koch LG, Britton SL, Davies KJ, Kouretas D, Wessner B, Radak Z. Resveratrol enhances exercise training responses in rats selectively bred for high running performance. *Food Chem Toxicol.* 2013 Nov;61:53-9.

Howatson G, McHugh MP, Hill JA, Brouner J, Jewell AP, van Someren KA, Shave RE, Howatson SA. Influence of tart cherry juice on indices of recovery following marathon running. *Scand J Med Sci Sports.* 2010 Dec;20(6):843-52.

Khan N, Mukhtar H. Tea and health: studies in humans. *Curr Pharm Des.* 2013;19(34): 6141-7.

Martinez-Gonzalez MA, Sayon-Orea C, Ruiz-Canela M, de la Fuente C, Gea A, Bes-Rastrollo M. Yogurt consumption, weight change and risk of overweight/obesity: the SUN cohort study. *Nutr Metab Cardiovasc Dis.* 2014 Nov;24(11):1189-96. Epub 2014 Jun 15.

Meyers K. What do pro triathletes eat for breakfast? Active.com. http://www.active.com /triathlon/articles/what-do-pro-triathletes-eat-for-breakfast. Accessed September 11, 2015.

Morihara N, Ushijima M, Kashimoto N, Sumioka I, Nishihama T, Hayama M, Takeda H. Aged garlic extract ameliorates physical fatigue. *Biol Pharm Bull.* 2006 May;29(5): 962-6.

Morris DM, Beloni RK, Wheeler HE. Effects of garlic consumption on physiological variables and performance during exercise in hypoxia. *Appl Physiol Nutr Metab.* 2013 Apr;38(4):363-7.

Nieman DC, Gillitt ND, Henson DA, Sha W, Shanely RA, Knab AM, Cialdella-Kam L, Jin F. Bananas as an energy source during exercise: a metabolomics approach. *PLoS One.* 2012;7(5):e37479.

Orlandi C, Tocco F, Concu A, Crisafulli A. Effect of beetroot juice supplementation on aerobic response during swimming. *Nutrients.* 2014 Jan 29;6(2):605-15.

Pinna M, Roberto S, Milia R, Marongiu E, Olla S, Loi A, Migliaccio GM, Padulo J, Shimabukuro M, Higa M, Kinjo R, Yamakawa K, Tanaka H, Kozuka C, Yabiku K, Taira S, Sata M, Masuzaki H. Effects of the brown rice diet on visceral obesity and endothelial function: the BRAVO study. *Br J Nutr.* 2014 Jan 28;111(2):310-20.

Pitozzi V, Jacomelli M, Catelan D, Servili M, Taticchi A, Biggeri A, Dolara P, Giovannelli L. Long-term dietary extra-virgin olive oil rich in polyphenols reverses age-related dysfunctions in motor coordination and contextual memory in mice: role of oxidative stress. *Rejuvenation Res.* 2012 Dec;15(6):601-12.

Rong Y, Chen L, Zhu T, Song Y, Yu M, Shan Z, Sand A, Hu FB, Liu L. Egg consumption and risk of coronary heart disease and stroke: dose-response meta-analysis of prospective cohort studies. *BMJ.* 2013 Jan 7;346:e8539. doi:10.1136/bmj.e8539.

Samaras A, Tsarouhas K, Paschalidis E, Giamouzis G, Triposkiadis F, Tsitsimpikou C, Becker AT, Goutzourelas N, Kouretas D. Effect of a special carbohydrate-protein bar and tomato juice supplementation on oxidative stress markers and vascular endothelial dynamics in ultra-marathon runners. *Food Chem Toxicol.* 2014 Jul;69:231-6.

Tsitsimpikou C, Kioukia-Fougia N, Tsarouhas K, Stamatopoulos P, Rentoukas E, Koudounakos A, Papalexis P, Liesivuori J, Jamurtas A. Administration of tomato juice ameliorates lactate dehydrogenase and creatinine kinase responses to anaerobic training. *Food Chem Toxicol.* 2013 Nov;61:9-13.

Womack CJ, Lawton DJ, Redmond L, Todd MK, Hargens TA. The effects of acute garlic supplementation on the fibrinolytic and vasoreactive response to exercise. *J Int Soc Sports Nutr.* 2015 May 14;12:23.

Yi M, Fu J, Zhou L, Gao H, Fan C, Shao J, Xu B, Wang Q, Li J, Huang G, Lapsley K, Blumberg JB, Chen CY. The effect of almond consumption on elements of endurance exercise performance in trained athletes. *J Int Soc Sports Nutr.* 2014 May 11;11:18.

Chapter 12

Damasceno MV, Lima-Silva AE, Pasqua LA, Tricoli V, Duarte M, Bishop DJ, Bertuzzi R. Effects of resistance training on neuromuscular characteristics and pacing during 10-km running time trial. *Eur J Appl Physiol.* 2015 Jul;115(7):1513-22.

Gilman MB, Well CL. The use of heart rates to monitor exercise intensity in relation to metabolic variables. *Int J Sports Med.* 1993 Aug;14(6):339-44.

Halson SL, Bridge MW, Meeusen R, Busschaert B, Gleeson M, Jones DA, Jeukendrup AE. Time course of performance changes and fatigue markers during intensified training in trained cyclists. *J Appl Physiol.* 2002 Sep;93(3):947-56.

Losnegard T, Mikkelsen K, Rønnestad BR, Hallén J, Rud B, Raastad T. The effect of heavy strength training on muscle mass and physical performance in elite cross country skiers. *Scand J Med Sci Sports.* 2011 Jun;21(3):389-401.

Luedke LE, Heiderscheit BC, Williams DS, Rauh MJ. Association of isometric strength of hip and knee muscles with injury risk in high school cross country runners. *Int J Sports Phys Ther.* 2015 Nov;10(6):868-76.

Madsen K, Pedersen PK, Djurhuus MS, Klitgaard NA. Effects of detraining on endurance capacity and metabolic changes during prolonged exhaustive exercise. *J Appl Physiol.* 1993 Oct;75(4):1444-51.

Muñoz I, Seiler S, Bautista J, España J, Larumbe E, Esteve-Lanao. Does polarized training improve performance in recreational runners? *J Int J Sports Physiol Perform.* 2014 Mar;9(2):265-72.

Navalta JW, Tibana RA, Fedor EA, Vieira A, Prestes J. Three consecutive days of interval runs to exhaustion affects lymphocyte subset apoptosis and migration. *Biomed Res Int.* 2014;2014:694801.

Neal CM, Hunter AM, Galloway SD. A 6-month analysis of training-intensity distribution and physiological adaptation in Ironman triathletes. *J Sports Sci.* 2011 Nov;29(14):1515-23.

Rønnestad BR, Ellefsen S, Nygaard H, Zacharoff EE, Vikmoen O, Hansen J, Hallén J. Effects of 12 weeks of block periodization on performance and performance indices in well-trained cyclists. *Scand J Med Sci Sports.* 2014 Apr;24(2):327-35.

Sedano S, Marín PJ, Cuadrado G, Redondo JC. Concurrent training in elite male runners: the influence of strength versus muscular endurance training on performance outcomes. *J Strength Cond Res.* 2013 Sep;27(9):2433-43. doi:10.1519/JSC.0b013e318280cc26.

INDEX

ABOUT THE AUTHOR

Matt Fitzgerald is an acclaimed endurance sports coach, nutritionist, and author. His many books include *Racing Weight, 80/20 Running*, and *How Bad Do You Want It?* Matt's writing also appears regularly in magazines and on websites such as *Women's Running* and competitor.com. Since 2001, his training plans have helped thousands of athletes of all experience and ability levels achieve their goals and he currently serves as a coach for BSX Athletics and Team Iron Cowboy. Certified by the International Society of Sports Nutrition, Matt has consulted for numerous sports nutrition companies and he is the creator of the Diet Quality Score (DQS) smartphone app. A lifelong athlete, he speaks frequently at events throughout the United States and internationally.